Tradition on the Move

Tradition on the Move

Leadership Formation in Catholic Health Care

Edited by

Laurence J. O'Connell and John Shea

MLC Press

Sacramento, California

Tradition on the Move
Leadership Formation in Catholic Health Care
© 2013 by Ministry Leadership Center

Published by MLC Press
1215 K Street, Suite 2000
Sacramento, CA 95814
916.552.2645
http://www.ministryleadership.net

Manuscript Editor: Robert Demke
Design and Composition: Catherine A. Hollingsworth and Brian O'Connell

ISBN 978-0-9887914-0-4
Printed in the United States of America.

This book is dedicated to the ongoing partnership among
the Ministry Leadership Center,
the Sponsoring Congregations of Religious Women,
the California Conference of Catholic Bishops,
the Alliance of Catholic Health Care,
and the leaders of
Daughters of Charity Health System
Dignity Health
PeaceHealth
Providence Health & Services
SCL Health System
St. Joseph Health

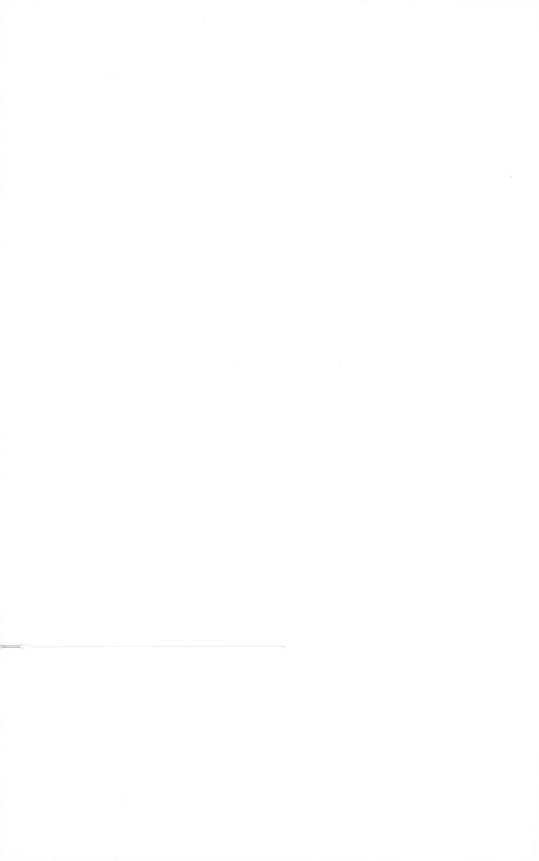

CONTENTS

The Restless Tradition

Laurence J. O'Connell and John Shea

Our hearts are restless until they rest in You.

—St. Augustine

Although the Catholic tradition has a justified reputation for conservation, it is also intrinsically restless. One source of this restlessness comes from its mission of bringing God's revelation to the ever-changing dynamics of time and history. The Ministry Leadership Center participates in this restive character of the larger Catholic tradition. We identify with the perspective of Pope Francis in his first homily: "Walking: our life is a journey and when we stop, there is something wrong." Thus, we focus our energies on the changing dynamics of leadership in Catholic Health Care, and we seek to provide ways to sustain the relevance and practical impact of the message of love and service within this ministry.

Our mission statement articulates this agenda: *The Ministry Leadership Center, grounded in the Catholic identity and tradition of its sponsors, forms leaders to sustain and deepen the ministry of healing.*

In the past, ministry leadership was largely entrusted to the women and men religious who established and directed our health care institutions. In recent years, however, leadership has been transferred largely to women and men who are not members of a religious community and who are indeed often not Catholic. This organizational transformation should be no cause for alarm. Understandably, though, the situation demands adjustment and a measure of recalibration. The tradition's natural tendency to read and adjust to the signs of the times is well suited to negotiating the curve into the future.

In response to the shifting terrain, the Ministry Leadership Center was established to bridge past practical wisdom with the lived experience of today's leaders. The Center invites leaders to cross the bridge, to enter new territory where the spiritual energies and practical demands of the tradition are integrated and gradually operationalized. The bridge is a three-year Leadership Formation program. Although everyone moves across at their own pace, the outcome is ideally the same—individual and organizational transformation.

Our vision flows directly from this transformative aspiration: *We seek to form a community of leaders who articulate and integrate a Catholic understanding of the ministry of healing.*

The Center serves as a meeting ground where individuals from a variety of personal backgrounds, professional experiences, and organizational affiliations create a shared identity and common understanding of the work entrusted to them. Building upon this foundational, enabling experience, participants report, almost without exception, a renewed and more gratifying view of their personal and professional lives. The assumption is that this positive energy will spill over into lives of the people who our leaders touch.

The Center's core values of *relevance, collaboration, and in-depth theology* guide the way we implement our mission and vision. The complexity and relentless pace of contemporary health care places extraordinary demands on leaders. The bridge between their day-to-day experience and the Catholic tradition must be uncluttered. Fortunately, the tradition is eminently practical. An informed yet pragmatic approach that values *relevance* is essential; the tradition's view of the human person as essentially social demands an emphasis on *collaboration*; and the ministry's grounding in the life and mission of Jesus requires access to an *in-depth theological* understanding of suffering and how we are called to alleviate, accompany, and transform it.

Tradition on the Move represents our reflection on eight years of experience with more than seven hundred leaders from six Catholic Health Care systems. We seek neither to make normative claims nor to suggest that we have the complete picture. We offer our experience and insights as a partial contribution to a much broader conversation. Ministry formation for twenty-first-century leaders requires reflection and experimentation on many fronts. The restless tradition of Catholic Health Care inspires us to always find better ways to care for one another. We are called ever forward!

ACKNOWLEDGMENTS

Ministry Leadership Center wants to thank everyone who has contributed to its origins and development. In particular, it acknowledges the singular work of its board and corporate members.

Alliance of Catholic Health Care

William Cox	2004–Present

Daughters of Charity Health System

Sr. Carol Padilla	2004–2005, 2009–Present
Fr. George Hazler	2004–2005
Stephanie Battles	2006–2012
Sr. Marjorie Baez	2005–2006
Julie Hatcher	2012–Present

Dignity Health

Christina Fernandez	2012–Present
Vickie Van Meetren	2012–Present
Sr. Brenda O'Keeffe	2004–2006
Rey Friel	2004–2008
Bernita McTernan	2008–2012
Charlie Francis	2007–2012

Members at Large

Bill Hunt	2010–Present
Darrin Montalvo	2010–Present

Ministry Leadership Center

Laurence J. O'Connell   2004–Present

PeaceHealth

Sr. Kathleen Pruitt   2010–Present

Carol Aaron   2010–Present

Providence Health & Services

Arnold Schaffer   2010–2013

Jack Mudd   2007–Present

Sr. Karin Dufault   2004–2005

Greg Van Pelt   2004–2009

Sr. Colleen Settles   2005–2009

SCL Health Systems

David Blake   2004–2005

Sr. Judith Jackson   2005–2010

Mary Jo Gregory   2010–2011

Irma Napoli   2004–2009

Terry Weinburger   2011–Present

Jill Willen Kennelly   2011–2012

Jason Barker   2012–Present

St. Joseph Health

Sr. Suzanne Sassus   2004–2008

Kevin Murphy   2011–2012

Jeff Thies   2008–Present

Sr. Jayne Helmlinger   2007–2011

Johnny Cox   2004–2006

Sr. Marian Schubert   2012–Present

Corporate Members

Lloyd Dean	Dignity Health 2004–Present
William Murray	SCL Health System 2004–2010
Robert Issai	Daughters of Charity Health System 2006–Present
Deborah Proctor	St. Joseph Health 2004–Present
John Koster, MD	Providence Health & Services 2004–2013
Michael Slubowski	SCL Health System 2011–Present
Bain Farris	Daughters of Charity Health System 2004–2006
Rod Hochman, MD	Providence Health & Services 2013–Present

In addition, we are grateful to Fr. Gerald Coleman for taking the time to read this manuscript and offering some helpful suggestions.

Conrad N. Hilton
F O U N D A T I O N

The Ministry Leadership Center gratefully acknowledges the wholehearted encouragement and generous financial support of the Conrad N. Hilton Foundation in preparing, publishing, and disseminating *Tradition on the Move: Leadership Formation in Catholic Health Care*.

Ministry Leadership Center
History and Conversation

Sharyn Lee, Laurence J. O'Connell, and John Shea

History

In 2002, William Cox, president and CEO of the Alliance of Catholic Healthcare in California, described the situation facing Catholic Health Care:

> *The most significant concern about the future of Catholic Health Care is that the hard realities being faced—depersonalized patient care, changing societal values, shortfalls in government payments, and culture-shaping market forces—have arrived at a time when there are ever fewer women religious available to help our systems and facilities develop effective ministerial responses. For nearly three hundred years, the Catholic mission in health care in the United States has been nurtured by thousands of religious sisters who founded and operated Catholic health care facilities and brought to them—in the words of the first president of the Catholic Health Association—"a spirit, a soul, an atmosphere and ideal of service . . . which they create[d] and maintain[ed] and [gave] their lives' best efforts to foster."*
>
> *Today, those culture-bearers are largely absent from the administration of Catholic Health Care organizations and less available for their governance. Without the pervasive presence of the sisters,*

1

the question is, how will the culture of Catholic Health Care be sustained and transmitted to the next generation of Catholic Health Care leaders? That culture, anchored in the healing mission of Jesus, is Catholic Health Care's raison d'etre—its meaning and purpose.Without it, Catholic hospitals may find themselves defenseless against the formidable threats to their religious identity and unable to continue as effective ministries of the Catholic Church.[1]

As a response to this concern, in October 2002, the Alliance of Catholic Health Care convened the sponsors and senior executives of the five Catholic Health Care systems with an acute care facility in California—Catholic Health Care West (now Dignity Health), Daughters of Charity Health System, Providence Health & Services, Sisters of Charity of Leavenworth Health System (now SCL Health System), and St. Joseph Health—and the Catholic bishops of California to examine these major challenges and to establish mutual commitments to address them. At this meeting the participants overwhelmingly identified an opportunity for collective action: "Developing and implementing a leadership program for formation with common foundations."

Founding the Ministry Leadership Center

Throughout 2003, a work group comprising representatives from each of the health care systems, the California Catholic Conference, and the Alliance of Catholic Health Care met to collaboratively develop the framework and business plan for a leadership formation initiative. In early 2004, the CEOs of five Catholic systems adopted the business plan and established and funded the Ministry Leadership Center (MLC). (In 2010 PeaceHealth joined the Ministry Leadership Center as the sixth sponsoring system.) The initial board of directors, chaired by Greg Van Pelt of Providence Health & Services and consisting of two representatives from each of the sponsoring systems, met to draft bylaws and articles of incorporation and to appoint a search committee. During these

---

Mission

The Ministry Leadership Center, grounded in the Catholic identity and tradition of its sponsors, forms leaders to sustain and deepen the ministry of healing.

Vision

To form a community of leaders who articulate and integrate a Catholic understanding of the ministry of healing.

Values

Relevance
To creatively link our work to the lived experience of the participants and to achieve our goals in a spirit of simplicity.

Collaboration
To foster active cooperation between and among our sponsoring systems, as well as other partners.

Theological Depth
To ground our work in Gospel values and the Church's core teachings.

---

foundational meetings, the board also established the Center's mission, vision, and values, and adopted the logo of a lodestar, based on the Mariner's Compass, which symbolizes a guide showing a way forward into uncharted territory.

After a nationwide search, Laurence J. O'Connell was invited to head the Center as executive director. In October 2004,

Dr. O'Connell addressed a joint meeting of bishops, sponsors, and leaders from the health systems:

> The Ministry Leadership Center is designed to create a community of health care leaders who will serve each other, who can depend upon each other as the ministry moves into some very demanding times. A common formation program will help create a shared vocabulary. It will develop a set of sensibilities that everyone will recognize and draw upon in hard times, and it will establish a network of lasting, supportive relationships. Ideally, we will create what my good friend Jack Glaser has called a "community of ministry" that "will be guided by an explicit and detailed understanding of the qualities it strives to deepen." We envision the emergence of a culture of community that might be reminiscent of—yet distinctively different from—the religious congregations we have known. The Ministry Leadership Center may well serve as an incubator where future forms of health care ministry and community may begin to emerge, a place where our leaders can lean into the winds of constant change and guide the Catholic health care ministry into safe harbor in the twenty-first century.

For the next several months, Dr. O'Connell consulted with the MLC board of directors to develop the program's expectations, requirements, logistics, and content based on the framework designed by the work group. John Shea was engaged as director of programs and processes development and Sharyn Lee became executive assistant and program coordinator.

Ministry Leadership Formation Program

The Ministry Leadership Formation Program, which was started in May 2005, is a three-year program that provides the working knowledge and skills to lead the ministry and mission of Catholic Health Care. Group One, comprising 120 senior executives from the five sponsoring health care systems, was divided into three "cohorts" of forty each. They met in three venues: Serra Retreat Center, Malibu, California; El Retiro Retreat Center, Los Altos, California; Palisades Retreat Center, Federal Way, Washington. Group Two, again comprising 120 senior executives, began in March 2006.

In early 2007, the three locations for the sessions were consolidated into one—Christ the King Retreat Center in Sacramento, California. This provided a uniform experience across all groups. In collaboration with Christ the King, MLC installed an up-to-date audio-visual system to enhance and capture the formation sessions. Group Three, with 120 new executives, began in November 2007 and the first group of participants completed their three-year program in February 2008. Since that time, a new group has entered the program approximately every sixteen months. To date, more than seven hundred senior leaders have completed or are currently involved in the MLC program. The seventh group of leaders will be welcomed in the spring of 2013.

Formation Integration Team

Besides designing and implementing a Leadership Formation Program, a complementary priority of MLC is to serve as a resource and consultant to sponsoring systems in the area of formation for their various constituencies. In November 2008, representatives of each system met in Orange, California, to explore a collaborative effort in the ongoing development and deployment of formation programs within the sponsoring systems, as well as to see how MLC could most effectively support them. This meeting led to the creation of the Intersystem Formation Task Force. The Task Force was charged with "taking into consideration the specific character, special needs, and particular organizational structures of each sponsoring system." This direction produced significant results and was succeeded by the Formation Integration Team (FIT).

FIT is an intersystem effort to support ministry formation within MLC's sponsoring systems. The team is a collaborative work group representing each of the sponsoring systems and is focused on:

- engaging system vice presidents of mission and formation in support of MLC participants and alumni, including clarity on expectations of MLC participants and alumni of MLC and within systems;
- collaborating across systems through the exploration of relevant common issues, identification of shared goals, and use of common tools to creating model practices and model templates for local adaptation; and
- sharing resources among systems via the web FIT resource library.

The resulting initiatives of FIT are anchored in an understanding of the "formation integration lifecycle" that incorporates careful attention to both personal and organizational development.

Alumni Formation

Closely connected to the work of both the Ministry Leadership Formation Program and the Formation Integration Team are the initiatives around ongoing formation for those who have finished the program. These initiatives include special offerings on the MLC website, reunion cohorts on concerns relevant to the distinctive challenges of the six sponsoring systems, an international cohort that makes a pilgrimage to the early settings of Christian Health Care in Turkey, and an intrasystem pilot on senior leadership formation.

MLC Staff Development

As the Ministry Leadership Formation Program and the Formation Integration Team developed, the staff expanded to meet the emerging possibilities. In 2007, Catherine Alesci became the program coordinator. In 2009, Mary Anne Sladich-Lantz joined the staff as director of formation integration, contributing to the design and implementation of program sessions. In 2009, Diarmuid Rooney was engaged as the director of integrated formation initiatives. He chaired the Intersystem Formation Task Force and developed the website as a program resource and intersystem learning platform. In 2011, Elizabeth McCabe joined the staff as director of system integration initiatives and leads the Formation Integration Team. In 2012 Kathryn Racine became project manager.

In 2011, three senior fellows were added to the staff. Andre Delbecq, who has contributed to the program from the earliest sessions, became the Center's senior fellow for spirituality and organizational leadership; William McCready, who has overseen evaluation and measurement from the beginning of MLC, became senior fellow for evaluation and strategic planning; and Bill Fitzgerald, who works with the MLC website and all technological services, became senior fellow for communities of practices.

Strategic Plan

The 2012 strategic plan for the Ministry Leadership Center has three goals. Goal One is to support program participants in the application of learned knowledge and skills in daily practice. Goal Two is to support the ongoing formation needs of the alumni as they emerge in each sponsoring organization. Goal Three is to serve as a resource and convener for intersystem collaboration. Under Goal Three there are two objectives: (1) demonstrate in practice the personal, organizational, and economic advantages of a collaborative approach to ministry leadership formation and (2) exhibit national leadership by encouraging the emergence of collaborative ministry leadership formation models. This book, *Tradition on the Move: Leadership Formation in Catholic Health Care*, helps realize the second objective of Goal Three. By publishing our efforts on ministry leadership formation, we hope to encourage and contribute to a national conversation on "collaborative ministry leadership formation models."

Conversation

In 2011, the Catholic Health Association (CHA) published its *Framework for Senior Leadership Formation*. The conclusion of that document traces the concern for leadership formation back to 1972 and cites the CHA publications that have contributed to analyzing and promoting that concern. It ended with a conditional hope:

> *Yet these efforts [documents on leadership formation] only take root and bear fruit when member systems take the initiative to develop this work in a way that recognizes both the commonality of our ministry across the nation and the unique cultural aspects of their respective systems....It is our hope that this resource will serve as a way to continue and deepen this important conversation, and translate that conversation into broader and more effective formation efforts.*[2]

Tradition on the Move: Leadership Formation in Catholic Health Care is intended to contribute to this conditional hope. We have done the work in "the unique cultural aspects" of our six sponsoring systems, and we recognize that what we have done could be relevant to the "commonality of our ministry across the nation." Now we want to "continue and deepen this important conversation" by reporting and reflecting on our experience in order to "translate [it] into broader and more effective formation efforts."

Formation Praxis

We began the Ministry Leadership Formation Program with some general ideas about formation, some convictions about how adults learn, and a sense that whatever we did had to have a real impact on the personal and professional lives of leaders, the people with whom they worked, and the mission of the organization.

With this blend of perspectives, we designed and began to implement the program. As staff, we were driven by MLC's values of relevance, collaboration, and theological depth that opened us to seek continuous quality improvement. As the program unfolded, this improvement came from both participants and presenters. Through their oral and written evaluations, participants became co-designers of the next steps. Presenters also evaluated what they did and what they saw happening and made suggestions. Staff, participants, and presenters developed the sense that they were in this together. We were convinced of the importance of what we were doing, even as we were discovering exactly what it was that we were doing.

Gradually, through our experiments in implementation, we developed some crucial theories about formation. Practice is the cauldron of theory. When we tried to put our theories into practice, their generalities were exposed and their certainties questioned. The rich particularities of actual situations resisted and nuanced what our minds had predicted would be relevant and effective. A dramatic way to frame this development might be that we came to a formation theory out of a formation practice. A more precise framing would admit that we had an intuitive sense of formation theory that was clarified, specified, and expanded by actually engaging in the practice.

> Through their oral and written evaluations, participants became co-designers of the next steps.

Therefore, our experience with formation falls into the category of praxis. We tried to put our ideas into action; and, in the course of those efforts, our ideas were changed. Then those changed ideas pushed us into new actions that, in turn, did the same thing that the first set of idea-driven actions did: they changed the ideas. As this dynamic interplay of ideas and actions continued, we became reconciled to the fact that it was not going to stop. This was just how it was. We were simultaneously spurred to refine the big picture of formation theories while we were refining the small picture of formation practices. Once we got the knack of praxis, the partnership of theories and practices seemed so interwoven that we could not do one without the other. Our only option was to cooperate with the process.

This praxis continues today. But we are at a stage where we need to ask anew and in a more thorough way a question we have asked before: "What's going on here?" We have decided to take the suggestion of Ronald Heifetz and Marty Linsky and distinguish the dance floor (action) from the balcony (reflection).[3] We have been on the dance floor. But we need the perspective of the balcony to become self-reflective and articulate what we have been doing. Of course, the purpose of the balcony is to study the patterns of interaction so we can return to the music and movement with renewed energy and direction.

Ministry Leadership Center Booklet

This is not our first time on the balcony. In 2011, we published a twenty-one-page booklet, *Ministry Leadership Center: Forming Leaders to Strengthen the Ministry of Healing.*[4] This booklet provides a brief statement of our program's theory and practice as well as a skeletal outline of its specific content. It was meant to be a quick, easy-to-read answer to the question, "What is the Ministry Leadership Center about?" It would inform anyone who was interested in formation about our approach. In particular, it could be given to sponsors and boards to apprise them about the formation experience of their executives, an experience that was often initiated and sustained by their decisions. Leaders could also hand the booklet to co-workers who wanted to know, "What exactly is this formation stuff?" The booklet was designed with these practical purposes in mind, and in our estimation it fulfills these purposes well.

For example, the nature and purpose of the program is concisely explained. The program is a three-year process that provides the working knowledge and skills to lead the mission and ministry of Catholic Health Care. The program is designed to nurture a community of leaders who genuinely identify with the Church's healing ministry, who appreciate its distinctive richness, and who are willing to commit to its long-term viability.

The formation theory and practice is succinct:

> *Formation is a process of socialization into the community and tradition of Catholic Health Care for the purpose of building up the community and carrying on the tradition. It begins by recognizing the established expertise of the participants in the diverse fields that comprise contemporary health care. These health care professionals are then invited into a formation experience that centers on the twelve foundational concerns that inform the distinctive identity and mission of Catholic Health Care . . . Vocation, Heritage, Spirituality, Responding to Suffering, Values Integration, Catholic Social Teaching, Clinical Ethics, Organizational Ethics, Discernment, Care for the Poor, Whole Person Care, and Collaboration with Church Authorities and Agencies. Throughout our program, we use the Triangle of Catholic Tradition, Cultural Information, and Individual and Communal Experience to develop the ability to articulate and integrate these concerns into the life and mission of their organizations.*

Finally, the formation experience is tersely described as creative, communal, and cumulative, and the content of the twelve foundational concerns is outlined in broad strokes.

Ministry Leadership Center: Forming Leaders to Strengthen the Ministry of Healing is a booklet that falls into the category of executive summary. It comprises headlines. But headlines need more extended stories if they are to be understood. It is a precise statement. But precision needs elaboration if it is to be appreciated. The booklet says it all in a few words. But when the few words are questioned and explored, more words inevitably come. It is time for MLC to express and communicate a more developed theory and practice of leadership formation.

Theories on the Balcony

When theories are identified and developed out of practices, they often come about because assumptions surface as we go about doing things; and once they surface, they beg to be elaborated. At least, this has been the way we have recognized our underlying suppositions and have begun the process of making them explicit.

In the course of doing formation, we found ourselves saying things like:

> *Well, in the Catholic tradition you are always going to have some resistance to the larger culture.*

> *Of course, this tradition values its heritage because it thinks something unsurpassed happened in the healing mission of Jesus.*

> *A tradition is always on the hunt for people to carry it on. Surviving through temporal passage is always an issue.*

> *The secular culture has trouble with theologically grounded ethics, and so it is not open to a lot of Catholic arguments. On the other hand, Catholics are always criticized for not making their arguments publicly available.*

> *You won't completely get this ethical position unless you grasp its theological grounding.*

> *The contemporary reflections on emotionally intelligent leadership are very complementary to what the Catholic tradition means by spiritual development.*

> *Ideas on participative management resonate with Catholic social teaching.*

Remarks like these are simultaneously tip-offs to submerged theories and invitations to take the time to surface and develop what is already present and operative. It is not a move from theories to practices; it is the discovery of theories within practices. However, it would be tedious and perhaps impossible to trace in a detailed way these connecting lines between existing practices and elements of theory. So for the purposes of order and communication, we will organize our reflection on our underlying theories about formation into four chapters.

Chapter 1, "The Meta-Story of Catholic Health Care and Leadership Formation," provides the ultimate framework for formation by portraying Catholic Health Care as a changing community that carries a founding revelation and creates developing traditions in interaction with a permeating culture. Within this framework, chapter 2, "The Process and Content of Leadership Formation," describes how organizational leaders are socialized into the community by gaining a working knowledge of the twelve foundational concerns of the tradition and by articulating and integrating that knowledge into their leadership activities, acknowledging that the final purpose of leadership formation is organizational transformation. These two chapters position and identify the work of formation.

Chapter 3, "Ministry Leadership Formation: Theological Grounding and Method," explores how theology is used in the process and content of formation. Since Catholic Health Care is a faith-based enterprise, it approaches whatever it does through theological rationales and motivations. This chapter explores how these theological perspectives can be introduced into the dynamics of leadership formation and how they can be used to ground organizational decisions. Chapter 4, "The Relationship between Leadership Development and Leadership Formation," connects leadership formation that comes out of the Catholic tradition with the ideas on leadership development that have been developed in the larger culture. Both chapters 3 and 4 develop critical ideas around two areas that inevitably appear in leadership formation—the place of theological perspectives and arguments and the incorporation of the competencies and strategies found in secular leadership development.

Practices on the Balcony

The same balcony reflection that clarified our theories refined our practices. Practice is akin to executing a strategy, and it is fraught with all the foreseen problems and unforeseen difficulties of getting something done. It is always an immersion into particularities; and no matter how prepared we are, particularities always bring surprises. Some spiritual traditions liken practice to counting seeds. It is meticulous work to organize details so that larger goals are achieved. However, for the purposes of this book, our concern is to find a way to express and communicate this demanding discipline of practice. How will we bring together the multiple activities that doing formation entails and recount the careful consideration that has be given to each of these activities?

We decided to divide formation practices into resources and adaptive challenges. This book will only deal with the adaptive challenges.

We have decided to distinguish formation practices into resources and adaptive challenges. "Resources" refers to the actual products we use in the formation sessions—leaders' workbooks, formers' guides, presenters' guidelines, power points, articles, input-exercises, process instructions for small and large groups, and so on. Although a few of these resources are referenced in the text and included in the appendices, this book will not deal with the specific content pieces of the program. We intend to publish a series of these resources as companion volumes to the present book.

In this book we focus on adaptive challenges. Adaptive challenges are situations and issues that accompany the effort of leadership formation. They are not isolated problems that can be solved and forgotten. They come with the territory of leadership formation; they are constant companions of programming. Chapter 5, "Adaptive Challenges in the Ministry Leadership Formation Program," identifies seven adaptive challenges—program content and sequence, presenters and staff, evaluation and measurement, off-site/on-site connections, adult learning method, system cooperation and collaboration, and alumni formation. It briefly describes five of these challenges and prepares the way for the following chapters that build on these descriptions and deal with three of these concerns in greater detail.

Chapter 6, "Evaluation and Measurement in Leadership Formation," provides a way to evaluate both programs and participants and develops analytic tools to assess leaders in terms of their working knowledge and skills of the twelve foundational concerns of the Catholic Health Care tradition. Chapter 7, "Formation, Technology, and Blended Learning," shows how technology connects the off-site and on-site worlds of leaders and strengthens community and integration. It also highlights the importance of web-based educational opportunities for contemporary formation. Chapter 8, "Facilitation/Resource in Leadership Formation," focuses on how adult leaders learn and the role of the facilitator/resource person in making that learning happen. Chapter 9, "System Cooperation and Collaboration in Leadership Formation," situates our Ministry Leadership Formation Program within the supportive context of each individual system and situates the individual systems in collaboration with one another. A reflection on "The Future of Leadership Formation" concludes the book with a series of programmatic and organizational considerations as well as a suggestion to adopt a specific attitude of hope that is indebted to the founding sisters.

Dialogue Partners

The fact that this book is praxis-generated means that it is not a normative book, proposing how formation *should* be done. It does not argue a case; it does not seek handbook status. It merely says: here is how we have done formation and here is what we think is important. We feel this limited ambition is appropriate because our purpose in writing is not to nail down a field. We want to become a dialogue partner, to enter into and contribute to the conversation on formation that the Catholic Health Association's *Framework for Senior Leadership Formation* hopes will emerge.

Who are the dialogue partners?

First, it is all those who are engaged with leadership formation in Catholic Health Care.[5] That would include the United States Conference of Catholic Bishops, bishops of individual dioceses, religious congregations, sponsors, boards, and leaders who have the responsibility for providing formation. It would also include leaders who are presently in or who have been through formation programs. Perhaps most directly, this book talks to people who are carrying out the formation imperatives of their organizations— mission leaders, educators, and so on. The praxis experience that has generated these reflections connects in an immediate way with all those who are designing and implementing formation programs and, in the process, finding themselves puzzling over theories and practices.

But the conversation is still larger. We are aware our leadership focus is very role-specific. Within Catholic Health Care, there are formation efforts happening with sponsors, boards, physicians, and the organization as a whole. Our concern with leaders is connected to each of these other organizational dimensions and can inform their programs; but each role also needs to be approached in terms of its distinctive contexts and responsibilities. Formation ideas that begin and develop in one organizational role can illumine and enrich programs for other organizational roles. But, most likely, they cannot be transferred into those programs without significant alterations. Of course, it is just this type of careful consideration that makes dialogue between leadership formation and other role formation both inventive and productive.

But the conversation is still larger. Catholic ministries as a whole are in a time of significant transition. It is recognized that this transition will only be successful if a formation process for future leaders accompanies it. This is especially true of ministries *ad extra*, those services that the Church offers to all people. Therefore, Catholic education on the primary, secondary, and higher levels and social service organizations such as Catholic Relief Services and Catholic Charities are seeking ways to sync their leaders to their missions; and a major way to do this is through leadership formation.[6] These groups might benefit from the experience of the Ministry Leadership Center and we might benefit from their experience.

Two further groups may be interested in what we have learned. The first is faith-based organizations other than Catholic ones. In today's world, all faith-based organizations are undergoing dramatic changes. These changes are needed for the survival of the organizations. But, given the nature of the changes that have to occur, organizational identity might be threatened. How will faith-based organizations continue to be Christian, Jewish, Buddhist, Islamic, and so on? Formation projects naturally arise in times of structural and attitudinal change.

The second group is those involved in leadership development in general. According to a good deal of organizational development literature, there is a contemporary crisis of leadership. What leaders have been about traditionally is not what leaders are called to be today. Many of the skills that got them where they are may not be the skills that the organization now needs to survive, adapt, and grow. In every sector of society, leaders have to engage in ongoing learning. The vision and skills they need to develop may be different from the vision and skills associated with Catholic Health Care formation. But both leadership development and leadership formation share the common ground of providing resources to ensure effective leaders. So a conversation may be mutually beneficial.

Finally, whoever may want to join the conversation, know this: you are welcome.

Notes

1. William J. Cox, "Sustaining Catholic Health Care as Ministry," address to the Leadership Conference of Catholic Health Initiatives, September 18, 2004.

2. Catholic Health Association of the United States, *Framework for Senior Leadership Formation* (Washington, D.C.: Catholic Health Association of the United States, 2011).

3. Ronald Heifetz and Marty Linsky, *Leadership on the Line: Staying Alive through the Dangers of Leading* (Cambridge, Mass.: Harvard Business Review Press, 2002), chap. 3, "Get on the Balcony."

4. This booklet has been distributed to the key personnel of the six sponsoring systems and to Mission and Human Resource leaders of other systems, as well as marketed nationally. For information on how to obtain it, visit our website at www.ministryleadership.net. Another earlier Ministry Leadership Center report was Laurence J. O'Connell and John Shea, "Ministry Leadership Formation: Engaging with Leaders," *Health Progress,* September-October 2009.

5. A particularly insightful dialogue partner is Catholic Health Alliance of Canada, *Forming Health Care Leaders: A Guide* (Ottawa: Catholic Health Alliance of Canada, 2009).

6. For the connection between leadership formation in Catholic Health Care and formation in Catholic higher education, see Andre L. Delbecq, Jack Mudd, and Celeste Mueller, "Formation of Organizational Leaders for Catholic Mission and Identity," *Journal of Jesuit Business Education* 3, no. 1 (Summer 2012): 57–73.

Theories

of the

Ministry Leadership Formation Program

CHAPTER 1

The Meta-Story
of Catholic Health Care
and Leadership Formation

John Shea

MLC came into the meta-story of Catholic Health Care through the mini-story of leadership formation. We had to construct and consult a big picture as we struggled with the decisions and details of the small picture. Big picture contexts are very appropriate to Catholic Health Care because it traces its identity back two millennia to the healing mission of Jesus and because its faith-based nature includes arguing from transcendent perspectives to proximate decisions and circumstances.[1] It is accustomed to seeing itself in the large light of historical passage and ultimate mysteries. Therefore, its natural language is meta (i.e., beyond, more, transcending, encompassing, and so on). Although some critics see this as a distraction from the demands of pressing situations and even as a substitution for action, faith-based traditions see it as putting in place a way of thinking that ensures fidelity to what really matters. Knowing the whole gives guidance to working with the parts.

We identify the whole as a "community and tradition" and see the two as so intimately interwoven that we often refer to them as community/tradition.[2] However, when we explore their depths, a more extensive set of historical and theological dynamics emerges. The community/tradition of Catholic Health Care is always carried

21

out within and in the name of the larger community/tradition of the Catholic Church. Within that larger reality the purpose of the health care community/tradition is to remember the founding revelation as the healing mission of Jesus and to carry and create traditions that embody that revelation as it intersects with culture after culture. The collection of these traditions (plural) becomes the Catholic Health Care tradition (singular), whose agenda is to be both faithful to the founding revelation and relevant to the current culture, while it witnesses to the deepest truths of Catholic faith. Throughout history, the health care community inherits, continues, changes, and develops its tradition.[3] Therefore, the whole of the health care ministry includes a specific way of connecting revelation, community, tradition, and culture. When these four categories inform and interact with one another, they tell the meta-story of Catholic Health Care. It is this meta-story that provides the ultimate rationale and inspiration for specific efforts of leadership formation.

Meta-Story

A meta-story is not a detailed history; and it does not substitute for a thorough account of what has happened or is presently happening. In addition, a meta-story does not deal with specific issues; and it does not substitute for problem identification, precise analysis, and effective strategy. Therefore, the meta-story is not an account of past events or an analysis of present problems. Rather, a meta-story identifies and describes the overall historical process, the perennial plot elements, and the dynamics that are always occurring. So no matter what happened in the past or is happening in the present, revelation, community, tradition, and culture are always co-happening. They are the structural constants and provide a framework for interpreting the ongoing events of Catholic Health Care.

There are important qualities to each of these structural constants. The revelation is founding. It is the origin, the genesis that is never forgotten, providing ongoing inspiration and direction, allowing the present activity of the Spirit to be discerned and engaged. The community is changing. If the founding revelation is to persist in and through time, the carrying community has to perpetuate itself, to find new people who will value and continue it. The tradition is developing. The people who carry the founding revelation are always encountering new situations and creating responses to those situations. These created responses become traditions that show the way caring for one another should be done. The culture is permeating. The founding revelation, the changing community, and the developing tradition exist within a larger, inescapable culture. The saturating influence of this culture affects every aspect of life and shapes how health care happens. Catholic Health Care has to determine what it wants to affirm, resist, and transform in this culture as well as how it wants to retell its story so that people in this culture will be able to hear and understand it. Therefore, the meta-story of Catholic Health Care is about a changing community who carries a founding revelation and creates developing traditions in response to a permeating culture.

> The meta-story of Catholic Health Care is about a changing community who carries a founding revelation and creates developing traditions in response to a permeating culture.

All four of these categories overlap with one another and each can be considered from the point of view of the others. Our concern with formation suggests that we begin with the changing community. It is the changing community that is inviting people who are already significant players in its complex work organization to become more involved with the community and more aligned with the tradition. It is the changing community that is remembering and consulting the founding revelation in ways that are appropriate to its current situation. It is the changing community that is preserving and adapting past traditions and creating new traditions that are designed to respond to contemporary demands. It is the changing community that interacts with the larger culture, embracing some aspects, resisting some aspects, and always seeking transformation. It does this even as it re-articulates its identity and mission in culturally relevant terms that allow the tradition to be understood and respected. Most of all, it is the changing community that will assess possibilities, make decisions, and wager on the way Catholic Health Care will continue in the future.

The Changing Community

The community of Catholic Health Care is grounded, sustained, and directed by the larger community of the Roman Catholic Church. This essential connection is captured in the phrase "Catholic Health Care is a ministry of the Church."[4] In this present time of significant change, new implications of this unchanging truth are being worked out. But the vital and necessary relationships between the Authoritative Magisterium, United States Conference of Catholic Bishops, local ordinaries, religious congregations, sponsors, boards, leaders, associates, physicians, and others are always in creative and collaborative interaction. Our concern is with leadership formation, and so we will approach these relationships from that point of view.

At the present moment, the community of Catholic Health Care takes the form of a complex work organization. It did not take this form in the past and it may not take this form in the future. In fact, throughout history it has survived and morphed many times, using different forms of organization to pursue its purposes. But in the United States in 2012, the community of Catholic Health Care is embodied as a complex and stratified work organization.

This thoroughgoing workplace character was reinforced when the sisters became employees.[5] Before the mid-1970s, religious congregations owned and ran hospitals, occupying key positions, from nurse at the bedside to president and chief executive officer. However, they were not compensated employees of the organization. Gradually, between the 1970s and 1990s, members of the religious congregation began to take salaries, apply for positions, and, at least in theory, compete with other candidates for those positions. There were many practical reasons for this development. But it was also a symbolic move. Now everyone in Catholic Health Care, excepting sponsors, boards, and volunteers, was a paid employee; and the ministry was conducted in and through, but never around, the dynamics of a workplace. Therefore, leadership formation into the community/tradition of Catholic Health Care takes place within the life of a work organization and has to respect those realities and take into account those boundaries.

Handing On

The key change in this work community is the numerical decline of women religious and their repositioning within the organizational structure. In the immediate past, they were significantly present in the delivery of health care. They not only sponsored the ministry and populated its boards, but they also were hospital administrators, department managers, technicians, direct care nurses, physicians, and so on. Over the last thirty years, the numbers of religious have been declining and their roles in the organization have been shifting. They are now mainly on boards and sponsoring groups. A widely accepted prediction is that very few religious will be involved on any level of Catholic Health Care in the near future.

> The key change in this work community is the numerical decline and repositioning of the women religious.

In the minds of many, this decline and repositioning of women religious threatens the identity of Catholic Health Care. Religious congregations have been the principal carriers of Catholic Health Care for centuries. The sisters have become so identified with

Catholic Health Care that it seems impossible to conceive of it without them. Therefore, when they are no longer a highly visible presence within the organization, the instinctive reaction is to question the catholicity of the operation. Can this be a Catholic hospital if there are no sisters or brothers walking the halls or in key administrative positions?

However, this is not the perception of the women religious themselves. As a general rule, they resist any over-identification of "Catholic identity and mission" with themselves. As one sister put it, "It was never about the sisters." Another sister chimed in, "Don't put the sisters on a pedestal." The sisters see themselves as servants of a revelation that has unfolded into a health care tradition. They have been the bearers of this tradition, but they are not the exclusive owners. What is important is that the tradition continues, that the torch is handed on to others. In Catholic ecclesiological language, the others go by the name of "laity."

Vatican II provided the grounding for this partnership and, in most cases, the eventual transition from religious to laity. Before Vatican II, religious and laity were often sharply contrasted. Religious had a special vocation and carried out specific ministries within the Church and special ministries on the border of Church and society like higher education, health care, and social services. The laity supported their work through prayer, financial contributions, and ancillary services.

However, the *Dogmatic Constitution on the Church* stressed a different type of connection.[6] Although there are diverse roles and responsibilities, a deeper unity bonds together religious and lay. All in the Church are called to holiness and all, by virtue of their baptism, are sharers in the apostolic ministry. The whole Church is called to holiness, mission, and ministry before individual religious vocations and the charisms of communities are taken into account. With this inclusive emphasis, there is nothing in principle against laity being essentially involved in ministries, especially those ministries on the border of Church and society. Therefore, it is not just the decline of women religious that brings laity to the forefront; it is a repositioning of the laity's participation in the life and ministries of the Church.

Division of Labor

As important as the willingness of religious congregations to partner and eventually hand over the health care ministry is and as helpful as the ecclesiological inclusiveness of the laity is in paving the way for this transition, these factors do not capture the extent or impact of the changes in the carrying community. First, the organizational leaders of Catholic Health Care are not exclusively Catholic laity. They come from and participate in other Christian denominations and other faiths. This means ecumenical and interfaith perspectives have to be explicitly acknowledged and taken into account. In this situation many think the faith grounding for leadership in Catholic Health Care is not only in the broadened ecclesiology of Vatican II but also in the Catholic social tradition, with its emphasis on people of good will, and in a developed theological anthropology that focuses on the common origin and destiny of humankind.[7]

Second, the division of labor of the immediate past has to be acknowledged as the starting point of change. The common perception and sometimes the explicit agreement was that women religious carried the mission of the organization and the non-religious carried the business.[8] This influenced hiring, advancement, and succession. The women religious hired both Catholics and non-Catholics primarily for their organizational and business acumen. Of course, these men and women who carried the business responsibilities also had to have a sympathetic connection to the mission. But since the sisters carried the mission, it did not seem urgent either to vet them from a mission perspective or, once they were hired, to form them in a mission perspective. Transecting the complex work community were two parallel populations on two parallel tracks, each with their own set of concerns and responsibilities.[9]

However, these parallel tracks did informally cross. Although it was rarely spelled out in organizational structures, many of the business leaders became quick and passionate learners and supporters of the mission. They grasped the Catholic ethos and saw its importance to the overall health care enterprise. Although mission might not have been part of their resume or their job description, mission became part of their heart. Although mission responsibilities rested with the religious, mission sensibilities were informally spread throughout the organization. When leadership formation finally arrived, the majority of leaders did not balk and ask why. They were open, ready, and even eager to learn and assume this responsibility, even if at times they felt intimidated by the challenge.

Nevertheless, the tracks remained in place and their differences became more apparent. While the mission track was losing its most prominent members, the business track began to increase in number. In the last thirty years, the business side of health care has become increasingly complex and competitive. To meet these challenges, Catholic Health Care hired more business people and expanded its organizational size. Partnerships, mergers, affiliations, and acquisitions also entered the picture. The result was a more imposing organizational and business presence whose importance to the survival of the organization overshadowed other considerations. Catholic Health Care, along with all for-profit and not-for-profit organizations, sought and paid for the best organizational minds. Criteria for successful businesses became the key factor in strategic decision-making; and the cultural way of doing the business of health care became, to a large extent, the Catholic way of doing the business of health care.

> When leadership formation finally arrived, the majority of leaders did not balk and ask why. They were open, ready, and even eager to learn and assume this responsibility.

This personnel scenario—a decrease in mission people and an increase in business people—carried the possibility of the business eclipsing the mission, the organization surviving but the identity lost. This possible mission eclipse is not directly intended. It is a side effect of the sheer volume and complexity of the business issues. It is presently estimated that somewhere between 60 and 65 percent of the people who work in health care never see a patient. Organizational overhead is daunting; and efforts to make it serve the delivery of health care are all consuming. Although there is sustained criticism of the bloated organizational structure of U.S. health care, for the present moment this is what it is and Catholic Health Care is part of it.

Catholic identity and mission may be lost or they may find new and more effective contemporary forms. It is this open future that pushes Catholic Health Care into the arduous task of becoming a formation organization.

Therefore, the community of Catholic Health Care is undergoing two waves of change. One wave is internal: the numerical decline and repositioning of the religious women who carried the responsibility for Catholic identity and mission. The other wave is the change in U.S. health care, of which Catholic Health Care is a part. This change has many facets, all of which have some impact on the range and content of formation. But the overall impact is the emergence of organizational bigness and business complexity. Both these waves represent dangers and opportunities. Catholic identity and mission may be lost or they may find new and more effective contemporary forms. It is this open future that pushes Catholic Health Care into the arduous task of becoming a formation organization.

The Formation Organization

Two initiatives drive the development of the formation organization. The first is the creation of mission positions in individual sites of care as well as in regional and system offices. Although the sisters cannot be replaced, particularly in their symbolic import, the role of keeper of the mission can be passed on; and the best way to do that is to institutionalize it. At the present time, the sisters hold many of these newly created positions. But the position descriptions themselves and the competencies needed for the position are not being developed with religious in mind.[10] The search will be for organizational leaders who can articulate the identity and mission of Catholic Health Care and integrate them into the complex, stratified work organization.

The second initiative, which intertwines with the first, is to have a formation component at every level of the organization—sponsors, boards, leaders, associates, those in direct patient care, attending and employed physicians, and so on. This is a very wide-ranging and complex undertaking simply because the work organization is very wide-ranging and complex. Formation efforts have to be shaped to particular roles and responsibilities. One size does not fit all. A formation program for sponsors cannot be the same as a formation program for leaders, and a program for leaders cannot be the same as a program for employed physicians. Yet all the formation efforts have to be aligned in some way so that Catholic identity and mission can be seen and enacted as a unity.

The level-related content and method of formation is closely related to the stratified structure of the organization. In theory, the higher levels of the organization see more of the whole; and their role is to express and communicate this vision throughout the organization. They are to bring this whole into the lower levels so that the work of all is appreciated and engaged from a unified and collaborative perspective. This visioning responsibility suggests that higher levels should have a greater degree of formation and advanced skills at articulating and integrating the whole into the parts. Lower levels need a lesser degree of formation. However, for formation to be calibrated along these lines, there is a need to clarify the distinctions and connections between all the levels. But, this type of stratified thinking is humbled by the universal experience of those in Catholic Health Care: workers at lower levels embody the mission and values to a greater degree than those at higher levels.

However, the challenge is more than just determining a different formational content and method for each organizational level. The ultimate purpose of formation is to recruit people to build up the community and continue the tradition. This recruitment naturally unfolds into questions of alignment, retention, and succession. In popular parlance, "Do they get it?" "Will they stay?" "Will the next ones continue it?" If people are not aligned but are retained, the community is not built up and the tradition is not continued. If people are aligned but not retained, the community is not built up and the tradition is not continued. If succession does not take into account alignment and retention, the community is not built up and the tradition is not continued. Therefore, there must be some favorable ratio of alignment, retention, and succession on each organizational level if the community is to be stable enough both to welcome new members and to continue the tradition.

> The ultimate purpose of formation is to recruit people to build up the community and continue the tradition. This recruitment naturally unfolds into questions of alignment, retention, and succession.

Beneath all the changes that the Catholic Health Care community is undergoing is a concern for the nature of the community itself.[11] To call workers a "community" connotes mutual caring for one another as the work is performed and the organizational goals are achieved; and this is a prime reason why Catholic Health Care calls itself a community. Catholic sensibility closely connects the ability to care for patients and families with the ability of the caregivers and the entire organization of which they are a part to care for one another. Only a caring community can care for others who come to them. But what form does mutual care take

31

in a complex organization where performance evaluations, firings, and downsizings are a regular and expected part? Compassionate care of patients is an overflow of a compassionate organization. But what does it mean to be a compassionate work organization?[12]

Organizational transitions, like transitions in personal life, combine grief and possibility.[13] The numerical decline of the sisters and perhaps their eventual disappearance from the ministry they shepherded for so long is painful. Even in these transitional years, when the writing of loss is on the wall, the sisters' combination of courage and care has been inspiring. In one of our sessions, we ask sisters from the six systems to give advice to the next generation of leaders. Along with encouragements to continue the Catholic identity and mission, each of the sisters said simply and directly, "Take care of yourselves." It was a telling and unrehearsed remark. They had cared not only for patients and families, but also for the people who cared for the patients and families. Above all, this is what should be continued and handed on—the spirit of caring that includes not only others but also yourself.[14] For the sisters caring was an affair of the heart. It radiated from their being and benefited all who came into their presence. To lose women of this spiritual magnitude is not an easy loss to bear. Grief is the appropriate response.

> Catholic sensibility closely connects the ability to care for patients and families with the ability of the caregivers and the entire organization of which they are a part to care for one another.

However, the other side of transition is potential. This potential is not unknown territory. The sisters had already explored it by sharing their vision with others and recruiting them into a life of service. What resulted were diverse levels of belonging and a division of responsibilities that worked together for the survival and excellence of the whole. This was present in the past as seed, and now it must develop into the future as tree. At the conclusion of our formation program, we recall the parable from the Gospel of Mark: "The mustard seed is the smallest of seeds. But, when it is sown in the ground, it becomes a tree and all the birds of the air make a home in it" (Mark 4:31–32).

This task of community continuance and development is accentuated today because multiple challenges are arriving from different directions—increased organizational and business complexity, significant shifts in reimbursements, the numerical decline and repositioning of religious women, a reordering of physician relationships, acquisitions and mergers resulting in new personnel, medical protocols that challenge compassion and dignity, societal pressures that are at cross purposes with Catholic mission, cultural antipathy toward faith-based operations, a secular consciousness that screens out religious motivations and rationales, a highly mobile workforce, and so on. But the task itself, the task of transitioning from one generation of Catholic Health Care leaders to another, is not new. Catholic Health Care knows its way around the vagaries of historical passage. After all, it audaciously claims that it goes back to the healing mission of Jesus.

The Founding Revelation

The changing community of Catholic Health Care identifies its founding event as the healing mission of Jesus and, in statement after statement, strongly states its commitment to continue the revelation that was present in that event. The general introduction to the National Catholic Bishops' *Ethical and Religious Directives for Catholic Health Care Services* (ERDs) begins, "The Church has always sought to embody our Savior's concern for the sick." The whole introduction builds on their earlier document, *Health and Health Care*, by citing Gospel examples of Jesus' care for the sick, a care that includes but goes beyond physical cure. It makes the further claim that the mystery of Christ illumines every facet of Catholic Health Care, and that Christian suffering and death can take on "positive and distinctive meaning through the redemptive power of Jesus' suffering and death." In fact, the Church's care for the sick throughout history has been done in "faithful imitation of Jesus Christ." This series of affirmations closely ties Catholic Health Care not only to the healing mission of Jesus but to the full revelation of the divine and human in Jesus Christ that the Church desires to hand on.[15]

The ancestry of Jesus is also reflected in the identity statement of the Catholic Health Association (CHA) published in 2001. This statement was the outgrowth of ten focus groups comprising more than one hundred "sponsors, system leaders, hospital and long-term care executives, mission leaders, system communicators, leaders from Catholic Charities, and heads of state Catholic health associations." The first sentence says, "We are the people of Catholic health care, a ministry of the church continuing Jesus' mission of love and healing today." The statement also refers to the "Gospel vision of justice and peace." Once again, the connection with the Jesus event is cited as the genesis of the Catholic Health Care tradition.

Although "continuing the healing mission of Jesus" is a special obligation of sponsors, it is a crucial piece of Catholic identity that is meant to inform the whole organization.

Individual systems and sites, connecting with the bishops and the professional society, refer to the healing mission of Jesus (or its variants). Each of our six systems connects with the founding Jesus event in their mission statement, in their values statement, or in other official documents. St. Joseph Health states its intention "to extend the healing ministry of Jesus in the tradition of the Sisters of St. Joseph of Orange by continually improving the health and quality of life of people in the communities we serve." SCL Health System carries "out Jesus' healing ministry today through [its] commitment to core values." PeaceHealth carries "on the healing mission of Jesus Christ by promoting personal and community health, relieving pain and suffering, and treating each person in a loving and caring way." Dignity Health is "committed to furthering the healing ministry of Jesus." Providence Health & Services remembers that "Jesus taught and healed with compassion," and the Daughters of Charity take "Jesus as [their] model." Although we do not have exact numbers, a reference to the Jesus origin is present in one way or another in many, if not most, Catholic Health Care systems.

This responsibility to "continue the healing mission of Jesus" is closely associated with sponsorship. The religious congregations have reconfigured sponsorship, changing membership requirements and explicitly working with canon law to ensure the juridical appropriateness of new organizational forms.[16] Although there is no one way that these new organizational forms are constituted, they do have a common mission. According to a collated summary from many sources, a key sponsor obligation is (1) to oversee, endorse, support, promote, sustain, ensure, and be accountable for (2) continuing, carrying on, extending, advancing, furthering (3) the healing mission of Jesus, the love of God manifest in Jesus, Christ's health ministry to people in need, the ministry of Jesus, Jesus' mission of love and healing, and so on. Although "continuing the healing mission of Jesus" is a special obligation of sponsors, it is a crucial piece of Catholic identity that is meant to inform the whole organization.

Rediscovering the Revelation

This commitment of Catholic Health Care to continue the healing mission of Jesus is not a way of dating and promoting an ancient pedigree. Rather, it is a startling claim: what happened in the beginning is relevant to what is happening today. But it even goes beyond that startling claim to affirm the presence of Christ today, not only to those who minister to the sick but to the sick themselves, who are accompanied and transformed in their suffering:

> *For the Christian, our encounter with suffering and death can take on a positive and distinctive meaning through the redemptive power*

of Jesus' suffering and death. As St. Paul says, we are "always car-
rying about in the body the dying of Jesus, so that the life of Jesus
may also be manifested in our body"(2 Cor 4:10).This truth does
not lessen the pain and fear, but gives confidence and grace for
bearing suffering rather than being overwhelmed by it. Catholic
health care ministry bears witness to the truth that, for those who
are in Christ, suffering and death are the birth pangs of the new
creation. "God himself will always be with them [as their God].
He will wipe every tear from their eyes, and there shall be no more
death or mourning, wailing or pain, [for] the old order has passed
away"(Rev 21:3–4).[17]

The full conviction of Catholic Health Care is not only that it
continues the healing mission of Jesus in time and space but also
that it is the sacramental and indeed real presence of Christ's
eternal work in the transformation of creation.

This deep truth of the spiritual presence of Christ drives Catholic Health Care to identify the historical continuities between
the healing mission of Jesus and the way we include and care for
the sick today. Whatever the discontinuities are, there are more
foundational lines of continuity. This is the basic intent of citing
origins as central to organizational identity and mission.Therefore,
it is necessary to articulate the lines of continuity as well as the
more obvious lines of discontinuity. It is also necessary to show how
these lines of continuity influence decision-making and strategies.
If this is not done, official written references to the importance
of this founding revelation become suspect.

At first, this continuity project seems to be a simple affair. We
have an intuitive and reflexive knowledge of our present situation; and we read the Gospels, the written witness to the healing
mission, from that perspective. We note a similarity of concerns
or values or purposes or situations. We articulate one or two
sentences that function as lines of continuity, a "thin" connection.

But the project of carrying a revelation through time and history is considerably deeper and more complex. It entails rereading the founding revelation in light of what is currently happening in both the tradition and the culture, and rereading the tradition and the culture in light of what is now seen in the founding revelation. When this happens, the thin connection is thickened; and the potential of the founding revelation to provide inspiration and direction is actualized. In organizational life, origin stories can become leadership tools to give the work meaning and the workers a sense of belonging.

However, since the "healing mission of Jesus" is a revelation, Catholic Health Care must continually be attentive to what it is revealing. As the community reflects on the healing mission of Jesus in light of the current state of the tradition and the culture, it comes to appreciate aspects that may not have been previously noticed. New meanings arise and they influence present directions. This capacity of the origin story is tied to the intertwined Catholic understanding scripture and tradition.[18] The scriptural account of the healing mission of Jesus always has more to tell us. As the community discovers this more, it re-articulates what the healing mission of Jesus means at this time and place. The community never pretends it has captured the whole revelation because its powers of comprehension are tied to its present historical moment. What it receives is like the coruscations of a turning diamond. While these flashes of revelation are not everything, they are what are needed here and now to continue the healing mission of Jesus.

For example, recently Providence, on the occasion of a reunification of Providence Services and Providence Health System into Providence Health & Services, reworked its mission statement. It had said: "Providence Health System continues the healing ministry of Jesus in the world of today, with special concern for those who are poor and vulnerable. Working with others in a spirit of loving service, we strive to meet the health needs of people as they journey through life." In a complex process that included all levels of the organization, the mission statement was changed to: "As people of Providence, we reveal God's love for all, especially for the poor and vulnerable, through our compassionate service." Providence rediscovered the revelation of the healing mission of Jesus and restated it as the ability of human love to manifest divine love when it manages to be a compassionate service to all, especially to those whose vulnerability might lead them to doubt they are loved. Their first and second mission statements are, on the level of words, two different statements. But, on the level of continuing revelation, they dwell within each other. The healing mission of Jesus is continued today where human love mediates divine love.

Other Catholic Health Care systems have rediscovered in the revelation of the healing mission of Jesus an emphasis on human dignity, the common good, diversity, inclusion, compassion, and so on. On the one hand, this suggests that the revelation is being retrieved through Catholic social teaching, which highlights these principles and states them in philosophic language. On the other hand, these discoveries reflect influences from the culture. They either affirm the best of what is happening in the culture or are an antidote to the worst that is happening in the culture. The founding revelation is always retrieved and restated in light of both the tradition and the culture.

> The founding revelation is always retrieved and restated in light of both the tradition and the culture.

Therefore, at the present moment, Catholic Health Care is in the historical process it has always been in. At the heart of this process is the important task of rereading the original revelation to discover its resources for contemporary challenges. When it does this, it acknowledges its debt to the healing mission of Jesus. It is from this source that Catholic Health Care brings forward love, dignity, diversity, and all the other principles and values it currently lives by. Continuing the healing mission of Jesus is not clinging to an outdated past. It is a creative dialogue with a revelation that understands and values the dynamics of how the deep mysteries of life unfold through the passage of time. The challenge is to understand and communicate these changes not as departures from the "healing mission of Jesus" but as articulations of that mission for this time and place.

The Unity of Catholic Systems

In the immediate past, most Catholic Health Care systems and individual hospitals identified their origins with the founding of the sponsoring religious congregations or with a specific missionary effort within the life of that congregation. The founders who were recognized, honored, and seen as imparting their spirit to future generations were people like Vincent de Paul, Louise de Marillac, Mother Joseph, Katherine McCauley, Emily Gamlin, Mary Potter, Mother Xavier Ross, Elizabeth Ann Seton, Jean-Pierre Medaille, and so on. These diverse origins underscored the differences among Catholic Health Care entities and promoted their distinctive charisms, the particular way divine grace was operative through that religious community. Women joined particular religious communities because of a "fit" between the charism of the community and their own gifts and talents. Charism was a discriminating factor marking differences.

> Although charisms are distinctive from individual to individual and from community to community, this distinctiveness is meant to identify contribution rather than celebrate difference.

In recent years, the communal nature of charisms has been stressed. Charisms belong to all in the Church and are developed for the benefit of all.[19] Although they are distinctive from individual to individual and from community to community, this distinctiveness is meant to identify contribution rather than celebrate difference. All the charisms come together for the common good. The theological grounding for this communal emphasis is the shared source of all charisms in the Spirit and their ultimate indebtedness to the founding revelation of Jesus Christ.

Therefore, when Catholic Health Care insists on a common origin in the healing mission of Jesus, it is repositioning the distinctive charisms of individual sponsoring congregations within this shared identity. Individual charisms are not lost, but their full potential is achieved in communion with the total gifts of the diverse members of the Church. The result is a better balance between unity and distinctiveness within the Catholic Health Care community.

This repositioning may have other advantages. It certainly supports doing formation across system lines and provides an ecclesiological rationale for the Ministry Leadership Center. But it also prepares the way for more extensive forms of cooperation. Many commentators think that only large systems will have the capacity to survive the social changes that are rapidly developing in health care, especially those that determine how the business of health care will be negotiated. If all Catholic Health Care entities arose out of a shared source, they have the required common ground for further collaboration. They should be open and ready to engage in the multiple ways of coming together that are available on the contemporary organizational menu—mergers, affiliations, joint ventures, acquisitions, partnerships, and so on. The healing mission of Jesus as the founding revelation supports the agenda of calling the full community of Catholic Health Care to work together in increasingly unified ways. If this greater collaboration happens, Catholic Health Care will consider it the way that the tradition develops in light of its founding revelation and cultural challenges.[20]

The Developing Tradition

There is an episode in the prehistory of Catholic Health Care that is instructive about how the community that continues the founding revelation creates traditions in response to situations in the larger culture.

In the early centuries of the Common Era, epidemics ravaged the Roman Empire.[21] They spread most quickly in the cities where there was overcrowding, limited water supplies, and poor sanitation. In the epidemic that raged from 165 to 180 CE, it is estimated that 30 percent of the population of Antioch died and another 30 percent fled, including the physicians. In fact, during this epidemic Galen, the most distinguished physician of this period, fled Rome. There was no dishonor in this. It was the accepted strategy.

However, Christians had a different approach based on a different reasoning. They believed God loved them and their response to this love was to love one another. "One another" meant all people, not just members of the Christian community. This was true in all circumstances. But when people were sick and possibly dying, it became the most urgent "place" for their universal love to be embodied. So when the epidemics came, the Christians stayed to nurse and care for the sick. They were living out their identity as loved and called to love.

Although no one is quite sure exactly what these ancient diseases were, modern medical experts believe that conscientious nursing cut the mortality rate. So when people who had fled came back to the cities after the plague had dissipated, they found many of their loved ones alive and well. Christians had nursed them back to health, combining courage and care. If their loved ones had died, Christians had been with them at the end and had buried them. They told the returning people how their loved ones had died and took them to where they were buried. Caring for the sick and burying the dead became Christian traditions.

These Christian traditions around caring for the sick and burying the dead complemented and corrected the dominant cultural behavior. Underlying this development was the motivational force of revelation. Christians had appropriated the spiritual vision of God loving them and they, in turn, loved one another. Spiritual visions always seek social forms for expression and communication. In response to widespread sickness and death, the traditions of caring and burying were developed and sustained. The meta-story of a community continuing a revelation and creating traditions in response to the permeating culture was unfolding.

Traditions and Tradition

This tradition-creating process continues with the passage of time. The result is an accumulation of traditions that eventually pressures the community into reflection and evaluation.[22] One concern is the relationship between the developing traditions and the founding revelation. The traditions make immediate sense because they are created as a response to present needs. The community naturally identifies with these creations and is known by others as people with these traditions.

However, the founding revelation may recede into the background. Although it was the motivational force behind the creation of the traditions, the traditions come to be appreciated and evaluated independently of their founding energy. For example, visiting the sick and burying the dead are respected as humane activities but their grounding in the dynamics of divine and human love does not accompany their ongoing development. Therefore, the community becomes vigilant in explicitly connecting the developing traditions to the founding revelation.

A second concern is the relevancy of the accumulated traditions to present situations. Traditions can be considered as the way the community does certain things. In Catholic Health Care this is how we welcome people who are not part of us, how we conduct our meetings, how we think about and deal with our finances, how we engage cultural positions we do not agree with, how we interact with political entities, how we understand death, how we relate to physicians, how we honor the best among us, how we deal with ethical issues, how we calculate wages, how we attend to grieving family members, and so on. This buildup of actions becomes "traditions," specific ways of thinking and acting in recurrent situations that have been around long enough to take on the status of how we do things.

With the passage of time, these traditions have to be examined. Some of them may still be relevant. Others may have become outdated. They were serviceable for the time in which they were created. But the times and consciousness have changed, and pruning is needed. Still other traditions embodied a false consciousness and had negative effects that were only gradually recognized. These traditions have to be eliminated. Other traditions were borrowed from the culture or imposed by the society. They have to be assessed in terms of how they fit with the identity and mission. In short, evaluating traditions is an essential activity as the meta-story of Catholic Health Care unfolds.

A third concern is the creation of new traditions to respond to societal and cultural developments. Today social and cultural change is rapid. There are new medical possibilities around genetic testing, emergency contraception, life-sustaining treatment, organ transplantation, and so on. There is new legislation around insurance coverage. There are new relationships with physicians. There are new cultural demands for diversity in the workplace. There is a need for more mergers, acquisitions, and partnerships in order to survive. Although the pace of these changes may slow or, what most commentators predict, increase, there will never be a time when the culture and society are not presenting new options. Catholic Health Care always was and always will be in a responsive position. The question is, how will the Catholic Health Care tradition welcome and evaluate these possibilities?

> As the community of Catholic Health Care moves through history, it carries both the founding revelation and the history of traditions that this founding revelation has generated, even as it creates new traditions.

Therefore, as the community of Catholic Health Care moves through history, it carries both the founding revelation and the history of traditions that this founding revelation has generated, even as it creates new traditions to respond to present situations. Sometimes this whole package is just called the "Catholic Health Care tradition." This use of "tradition" in the singular is meant to include the founding revelation and its plural traditions. In other words, it signifies the complete history of how Catholic Christians have responded to health and sickness. In this language, the acceptable parlance is that the community carries and continues the Catholic Health Care tradition. This tradition constitutes its identity and becomes a resource in meeting present and future demands. As the community confronts new situations, it reaches into its tradition and brings forward what it needs. To grasp the full extent of the Catholic Health Care tradition as a resource, it is necessary to position this tradition within the larger Catholic tradition of which it is a part.

Catholic Tradition

The phrase "Catholic tradition" connotes the whole of Catholic Christianity. It includes the founding revelation in all its completeness (not just the healing mission of Jesus), and all the ways that revelation has been explained and expanded throughout the centuries. Within the Catholic tradition there are multiple sub-traditions—liturgical, ascetical, dogmatic, moral, ministerial, educational, and so on. Catholic Health Care is one of these sub-traditions, and this status is often expressed in the phrase "Catholic Health Care is a ministry of the Church." [23] The larger reality of the Church has a health care ministry, supplying inspiration and direction to its efforts. In organizational terms, Catholic Health Care's relationship with the Catholic tradition brings it into dialogue and collaboration with the local bishop, the United States Conference of Catholic Bishops, canon law, larger Church structures, and higher levels of authority.

In principle, the community/tradition of Catholic Health Care can call on everything within the Catholic tradition. Some see this connection in terms of inheriting and sharing certain Catholic characteristics. For example, Catholic Christianity has a sacramental sensibility, a community emphasis, a great respect for authority, a high evaluation of human rationality, a central place for charity, a preferential option for the poor, a belief in the essential dignity of the person, and so on. These characteristics describe a Catholic ethos that distinguishes Catholic Christianity from other Christian traditions. It is assumed these characteristics are expressed in one way or another in every Catholic enterprise. So one way Catholic Health Care is embedded in the Catholic tradition is through the presence of these characteristics in its mission and operations.

However, there is also a more concrete and discerning connection. Catholic Health Care selectively chooses from the resources of the larger Catholic tradition. For example, in the larger Church world there are current conversations around access to priesthood and diaconate, the doctrinal content of religious education textbooks, changes in liturgical language, approved biblical translations, the status of national hierarchies, sexual abuse scandals, evangelization efforts, and so on. These discussions have little impact on health care; and, for the most part, the community of Catholic Health Care does not enter into them or draw on them to carry out its ministry.

But other concerns of the larger Catholic tradition are more relevant. The conversations around interfaith dialogue and cooperation are germane to a ministry that is carried out by an interfaith workforce and serves an interfaith patient and family population. Since Catholic Health Care is always dealing with permissible and impermissible medical procedures and discerning what partnerships and affiliations are appropriate, the moral theology around medical and organizational ethics is always relevant. Catholic Health Care has a special relationship with the local ordinary, so how bishops are appointed to particular dioceses is always on the radar screen of sponsors, boards, and leaders. The Catholic discussion on the relationship of priesthood to lay ecclesial ministries affects who will and will not be called chaplains in health care settings. Since Catholic Health Care is an American workplace, the principles of Catholic social teaching are immediately applicable. Most recently, even the spirituality strands of Catholicism have become relevant as cultural movements advocate for the spiritual development of leaders and workers. More connections to the larger Catholic tradition could be cited, but the basic observation remains: The community/tradition of Catholic Health Care reflects some strands of the Catholic tradition more than others. It carries the Catholic agenda, but not the whole Catholic agenda in an overt way.

Catholic Identity and Mission Today

When Catholic Health Care is appreciated as a tradition, there is a strong sensitivity to historical passage. It is coming from the past and going to the future, and the challenge is to manage the transition. This challenge includes re-articulating Catholic identity and mission for the present time. MLC, in dialogue with the Catholic Health Association and Catholic Health Care organizations throughout the United States, describes the present identity and mission of the tradition in terms of twelve foundational concerns: Vocation, Heritage, Spirituality, Responding to Suffering, Values Integration, Discernment, Clinical Ethics, Organizational Ethics, Catholic Social Teaching, Care for the Poor, Whole Person Care, and Collaboration with Church Authorities and Agencies.[24] Taken together, these concerns capture the knowledge that must be handed on from one generation to the next.

However, identifying these twelve concerns should not give the impression that the tradition has a finished form, an isolated and self-enclosed identity. These concerns have surfaced because of the tradition's ongoing interaction with past and present cultures. In fact, the influence of the contemporary culture is so strong that it shapes how these concerns are understood and implemented. The loud and insistent voice of the culture forces a conversation that influences every aspect of the changing community, the founding revelation, and the developing tradition. In short, the culture is permeating.

The Permeating Culture

Although the community/tradition strongly differentiates itself from the larger culture, a complete separation is never achieved. The larger culture generates social forms that everyone has to deal with and creates a consciousness that everyone has to negotiate. Therefore, the Catholic tradition in general and the Catholic Health Care tradition in particular struggle to develop a nuanced relationship to the larger culture.

Affirmation, Resistance, Transformation

The first and most fundamental move of the community/tradition toward the culture is to affirm what is positive and to participate in it. The potential for this affirmation comes from two distinctive theological perspectives of the Catholic tradition. First, the dynamics of divine grace and human cooperation are coextensive with creation. So what people have created in any place and time can be genuine contributions to the ongoing improvement of the human community. Second, the Holy Spirit is present with the Church as it moves through history; and so its developments over time can be appreciated as steps toward fulfillment. Since these developments unfold in interaction with culture, the culture can be appreciated as a graced collaborator in the Church's mission. Therefore, the basic stance of the community/tradition toward the culture is appreciation and openness.[25]

This affirmation stance of the community/tradition is usually just assumed. Catholic Health Care pursues the legitimate cultural advances of medicine, embraces the cultural consumption of technology, cooperates with culture-wide initiatives in health care, receives grants from cultural foundations, administers government-funded social programs, and so on. However, it may both participate in these cultural activities and harbor hesitancies for different reasons and from different motivations.[26]

Resistance, the more publicized face of the community/ tradition toward the culture, often overshadows the stance of affirmation. There are many assumptions, structures, policies, perspectives, and practices that the larger culture either encourages or permits that contradict the convictions and values of the community/tradition. Since the larger culture defines the smaller entities within it by their compliance or non-compliance with its dictates, Catholic Health Care becomes identified with its points of resistance and pressured to conform. What Catholic Health Care will not go along with becomes, in popular consumption, what Catholic Health Care is. Therefore, the ability to situate resistance within the meta-story of Catholic Health Care and to effectively express and communicate the reasons for the resistance is crucial.

As the stance of affirmation is theologically grounded, so is the stance of resistance. If people are free to cooperate with divine initiatives and contribute to human well-being, they are also free to refuse to cooperate with those initiatives and create structures and behaviors that jeopardize human well-being. The Catholic tradition has a stubborn insistence on freedom and the corresponding responsibility to discern right from wrong and to act accordingly. Therefore, ethical discernment, grounded in theological convictions, accompanies every step of Catholic Health Care's strategic decision-making. There will always be some assumptions Catholic Health Care will not embrace, some behaviors it will not condone, some laws it will not tolerate, some policies it will not endorse, and so on. The "yes" of affirmation is balanced by the "no" of resistance. In contemporary health care, this translates into the legal arena of first amendment rights and conscience clauses.[27]

A third stance develops out of the combination of affirmation and resistance. In the self-understanding of Catholic Health Care, the community/tradition is not meant to be absorbed in its own struggle to survive. Its mission is to be a seed of transformation in the larger culture. It calls the culture to persist in the paths that maximize human well-being and models a way of serving that is meant to show the true potential of every human being and community. The self-understanding of the Church is that it has something valuable to give to society, something that the society is already looking for but has not yet found.

Therefore, the larger culture must be engaged and challenged in those areas where it has to change, where how it presently operates ignores or undercuts the potential for a better world. In the theological language of the Catholic tradition, the purpose of the Church is the Kingdom of God, the transformation and fulfillment of all creation. Therefore, Catholic Health Care will always advance an agenda larger than its own internal concerns, asking itself how it is contributing to the ongoing emergence of what God is calling creation to become. It is this theological motivation that pushes Catholic Health Care into the arena of political advocacy and social change.

These stances of affirmation, resistance, and transformation in relation to the larger culture are basic orientations, predictable ways of relating. They are fleshed out through specific issues.

These stances of affirmation, resistance, and transformation in relation to the larger culture are basic orientations, predictable ways of relating. They are fleshed out through specific issues. But the community/tradition is particularly sensitive to one aspect of the larger culture that permeates every issue. This aspect is atmospheric, a mood that always has to be respected because all thought and action has to be cast in its categories. If it is not, the majority of people, both within and outside the Church, will not understand it. So even as it is resisted on one level, as it has to be, it must be engaged on another level. The larger culture is secular.[28]

Integral Humanism

More appropriately said, the mood of the larger culture is secular humanism.[29] It focuses on the physical, social, and mental dimensions of human experience, explores those dimensions at great length, and suggests strategies to be intentional about them. This focus monopolizes consciousness, restricting attention to bodily health and sickness, relational well-being among family and friends, the demands of work and personal life, the interaction of societal groups, and, especially, swings in economic security. These facets of life have to be addressed and mature living struggles to find a way for everyone to prosper as they are held together. This single-mindedness and sustained focus have benefited a wide range of humanistic endeavors. In particular, it has contributed to medical advances and innovations in the delivery of health care.

However, from the point of view of Catholic Health Care, the mood of secular humanism has a serious deficit. Secular humanism excludes the spiritual dimension or merely tolerates it, relegating it to a private matter and categorizing it as individual quirkiness.[30] Although there are explicit branches of atheism within secular humanism, for the most part secular humanism simply ignores the subtler sensitivities of spirit or conflates them with mental states and attitudes. It also disregards ultimate questions as unsolvable and irrelevant. Instrumental reasoning rules and mystery, especially the ultimate mystery of life, is not taken into account. In the grip of this mood, leaders become "uncomfortable" with spirituality, especially God language, and often become visibly irritated when theological contexts and their derived ethical considerations are discussed. Work life is solving problems or adjusting to chronic adaptive challenges. Spiritual considerations are too vague and deeper questions are not immediately relevant.

This mood threatens ways of articulation that have been key to Catholic Health Care. As a faith-based enterprise, Catholic Health Care has been explicitly theological in both its individual motivations and its public rationales. Religious men and women and other key leaders have been personally driven by some variant of love of God and neighbor that is at the heart of Christianity. When pushed to say why they were dedicating their lives to Catholic Health Care, they would reach beyond social reasons into spiritual perceptions and theological motives. If they were pushed to explain organizational decisions and policies, they would mention faith convictions and values as well as point out the social benefits. The secular mood's diffidence in regard to ultimate motivations for leaders and ultimate rationales for organizations entails a serious loss of identity-generating language for Catholic Health Care.

Of course, Catholic tradition and Catholic Health Care challenge this mood and its reductionist tendencies. As important as advances are in physical, social, and mental life, an exclusive focus on these dimensions truncates the full human condition. But it is not enough to issue denunciations of secular humanism. Since Catholic Health Care is a sub-tradition that lives on the border of Church and society, secular humanism is both a dialogue partner and a point of view that is deficient from the viewpoint of religious traditions.[31]

Therefore, in response to secular humanism, the Catholic tradition has "talked back" with integral humanism or true humanism or authentic humanism.[32] This idea adds the missing spiritual and theological component and articulates it in such a way that it contributes to the flourishing of what secular humanism is most concerned about—physical, social, and mental life. The humanism of secularity is included and transcended by the inclusiveness of the Catholic tradition and the Catholic Health Care tradition.

Integral humanism reinterprets and repositions Catholic Health Care's appeals to spirituality. Spirituality is appreciated as a resource for human development, emphasizing how it suffuses and elevates mental and social activities with passion and creativity. The Catholic tradition has documented this enhancing quality of spirituality by identifying twelve fruits and seven gifts of the Spirit, all of them forms of human excellence.[33] In a broader sense, Spirit was always presumed to be present when the mind was illumined, the will was inspired, and the heart was gladdened. Spirituality is not in competition with human development; it is its deepest energy and most perseverant force.[34]

Integral humanism also reinterprets and repositions Catholic Health Care's appeals to theology. Theological convictions function as the grounding for the guiding values and the desired behaviors of the organization.[35] Although individual leaders will anchor the values in their own experiences and beliefs, Catholic Health Care, as a faith-based enterprise, grounds the values in explicit theological convictions. The Catholic tradition is rational; and Catholic Health Care exhibits that rationality when it argues that its values spring from the real relationship between the divine source and humanity. Theology answers the question of ultimate rationale: "Why are we doing this?" This question often arises when the mission is difficult and commitment is wavering. When theology works, it creates meaning that reinvigorates a course of action. It ties the question of God to the questions we have about ourselves.[36]

In response to secular humanism, the Catholic tradition has "talked back" with integral humanism or true humanism or authentic humanism.

Catholic Health Care lives out of its own traditions. But these traditions are formed and reformed in relationship to culture, and there are predicable dynamics to that relationship. The Catholic tradition will always be predisposed to affirm, resist, and transform aspects of the culture. But it will also heed the cultural mood and develop a language that is current and relevant to it as well as part of its own history. This is what is happening with spirituality and theology, two essential components of the Catholic Health Care tradition. Spirituality is a resource and theology is the grounding for maintaining and advancing the identity and mission of Catholic Health Care.

Today

This meta-story is able to predict how Catholic Health Care will behave. Wherever Catholic Health Care has been and wherever it will be, it is a changing community that carries a founding revelation and creates developing traditions in interaction with a permeating culture. This ultimate frame is a generous house. It has room for all kinds of complementary and even contradictory analyses of Catholic Health Care—psychological, social, political, economic, medical, religious, and so on. It can absorb and respond to whatever comes its way. So what is happening today, both positively and negatively, becomes another chapter in the story we know and are presently living.

The meta-story also makes the current agenda clear. Any enterprise that wants to survive over time must be attractive enough and entrepreneurial enough to recruit new people into its service. This must be so much a part of its modus operandi that recruitment is on an equal footing with the provided services. In fact, the people and the services are so intimately linked, so interdependent with one another, that it is impossible to conceive of the services without conceiving of people who are formed in a certain way to provide them. Quite simply, Catholic Health Care is looking for the right people.[37]

Sometimes there is a match between the community/tradition and the culture that supports finding the right people. There is nothing automatic about discovering this common ground. It often begins as an intuition that may or may not develop positively. It is a possibility that has to be carefully and thoughtfully explored. But there is enough initial recognition for further conversation to be pursued. At MLC, we believe this incipient mutuality is present today. There is a symbiotic relationship between the Catholic Health Care formation agenda and the desires of American workers.

According to many commentators, American workers are extending their expectations.[38] When people are searching for work, there is always the drive for the highest salary and the best benefits. But this drive has been joined by the desire for positive workplace relationships and meaningful work. In fact, there are some indications that people seek out faith-based organizations because they expect relationships and meaning to be part of the workplace culture. When formation is seen as socialization into the community/tradition of Catholic Health Care, it plays into these desires. Whatever else formation does, it definitely strives to maximize work relationships and heighten the sense of contribution to the common good. These are important ways in which meaning is achieved. What formation offers is what many workers may want.

For us, this is a partial explanation for why the leaders who come into the program are so highly motivated and interested. Whether the leaders are Catholic or non-Catholic, there is little or no resistance to the idea of taking a deeper look into the identity and mission of the organization. They have been part of this organization and have risen in its ranks. There may have been some informal and even formal formation along the way. But now seems an appropriate time for a deeper dive. So, as our succinct statement says, they are invited into a "formation experience that centers on the twelve foundational concerns that inform the distinctive identity and mission of Catholic Health Care."

Notes

1. For an understanding of the historical nature of the Catholic Church that also, in some respects, extends to the sub-tradition of Catholic Health Care, see the Second Vatican Council's *Dogmatic Constitution on the Church*, chap. 2, "The People of God." In this chapter, the Church is examined through the lens of both its passage through time and its extension throughout the world.

For an understanding of how arguments from transcendent convictions are conducted, see the Second Vatican Council's *Pastoral Constitution on the Church in the Modern World*, chap. 2, "The Community of Mankind." In this chapter, the theologically grounded common origin and destiny of humankind is used to critique vast economic disparity in the social order. This critique leads to a call for a more equitable distribution of the goods of the earth. This argument is common in Catholic social teaching. Both documents are available in Austin Flannery, OP, ed., *Vatican Council II: The Conciliar and Post Conciliar Documents,* new rev. ed. (Northport, N.Y.: Costello Publishing; Grand Rapids, Mich.: William B. Eerdmans, 1992).

2. Our succinct statement reads: "Formation is a socialization process in the community and tradition of Catholic Health Care for the purpose of building up the community and carrying on the tradition."

3 For an understanding of the essential characteristics of tradition and how these characteristics are deeply challenged by modernity, see Langdon Gilkey, *Catholicism Confronts Modernity* (New York: Seabury Press, 1975), chap. 3, "Sources and Tradition."

4. Of course, both women religious and brothers have carried the identity and mission of Catholic Health Care. But congregations of women religious sponsor our six systems and we reference this immediate situation.

5. See the *Dogmatic Constitution on the Church*, chap. 4, "The Laity." For the post-conciliar development of the intra-Catholic understanding of the laity with a special reference to Catholic Health Care, see Zeni Fox, "Making All Things New: Catholic Health Care, The Laity, and The Church," *Health Progress*, September-October 2011.

6. These issues will be addressed in chapter 3, "Ministry Leadership Formation: Theological Grounding and Method."

7. This distinction between mission and business (mission and margin) is common in Catholic Health Care and can be understood in different ways. Sometimes it is characterized as two different sets of activity. Mission involves spirituality, ethics, pastoral and spiritual care, and so on, and business involves the financial, legal, and organizational aspects of health care delivery. However, we prefer to distinguish un-integrated mission and business from integrated business and mission. The two can be distinguished in the following way.

The complex work organization, which is shaped by governmental regulations, economic pressures, and societal strictures, is the common form of U.S. health care. Catholics, along with everyone else, adopt and work within this form. If this form and its default ways of operating are taken over without vetting them through the ethos of Catholic Health Care, mission and business are not integrated. They become two parallel tracks. The resulting impression is that Catholic Health Care is Catholic in name only because it actually operates like everyone else. Since no one can see a difference in structures and behaviors, the mission is relegated to the realm of ineffective motivation.

However, if the commonly shared cultural form is vetted through the ethos of Catholic Health Care, then the form is affirmed, changed, and developed in light of the Catholic identity and mission. This vetting is sometimes called "baptizing" a cultural form. One of the goals of formation is to provide leaders with the ability to engage in the ongoing process of mission integration, allowing the Catholic ethos to inform and transform the default way of health care operations that are inherited from the larger culture.

8. See John O. Mudd, "From CEO to Mission Leader," *America* 193, no. 2 (July 18, 2005).

9. See the mission competencies developed by CHA, www.chausa.org/missionleadercompetencies.

10. A helpful way to conceptualize an organizational community is to position it between primary group and formal association. In a primary group mode, people relate face-to-face and include issues of personal well-being. In an association mode, people relate to one another through role requirements and responsibilities. A community mode swings between primary group relating and association relating. The community discerns when the mutual concern of the group for one another should be attended to and when the role-structured work should be the focus. Evelyn Eaton Whitehead and James D. Whitehead, *Community of Faith: Crafting Christian Communities Today* (New London, Conn.: Twenty-Third Publications, 1992), esp. chap. 2, "Community Is a Way to Be Together."

11. For insights into how organizations become compassionate, see www.compassionlab.com.

12. William Bridges, *Managing Transitions: Making the Most of Change* (Cambridge, Mass.: Da Capo Press, 1991).

13. In the last analysis, it may be the ability to create a caring organization that is at the core of handing on the tradition. Barbra Mann Wall reports on interviews with Sr. Sheila Lyne of Mercy Hospital and Medical Center in Chicago and Sr. Carol Keehan, president of Catholic Health Association, that "they and other sisters and brothers understood what many lay corporate managers failed to grasp: that in the business of serving people, it is people themselves that ultimately matter most—not dollars or margins or numbers, but acknowledging individuals' needs, being kind and accessible, and in short, caring more about them than about the business that serves them. To the extent that these values can prevail in modern Catholic hospitals, these hospitals' impact on U.S. medical culture will remain strong, regardless of the diminishing number of sisters and brothers who walk their halls or fill their boardrooms." Barbra Mann Wall, *American Catholic Hospitals: A Century of Changing Markets and Missions* (New Brunswick, N.J.: Rutgers University Press, 2011), 180.

14. Vatican II, *Dogmatic Constitution on Divine Revelation*, chap. 2.

15. For a secular point of view that explores how origin stories continue in the ongoing life of organizations, see Michael S. Poulton, "Organizational Storytelling, Ethics, and Morality: How Stories Frame Limits of Behavior in Organizations,"

Electronic Journal of Business Ethics and Organization Studies 10, no. 2 (2005): 4–9; Jim Collins, *Good to Great* (New York: HarperBusiness, 2001), esp. chap. 9, the discussion of preserving the core while changing practices and strategies; and Peg Neuhauser, *Corporate Legends and Lore: The Power of Storytelling as a Management Tool* (New York: McGraw-Hill, 1993), esp. chap. 5, "Your Corporate Heritage: Sacred Bundle Stories."

16. See Mary Kathryn Grant and Sister Patricia Vandenberg, "After We're Gone: Creating Sustainable Sponsorships," in "Sponsorship: Our Enduring Link," special issue, *Health Progress,* January-February 2007; and the section on "Sponsorship" on the Catholic Health Association website.

17. "General Introduction," *Ethical and Religious Directives for Catholic Health Care Services.*

18. "Sacred Tradition and sacred Scripture, then, are bound closely together, and communicate one with the other. . . . Hence, both Scripture and Tradition must be accepted and honored with equal feelings of devotion and reverence." *Dogmatic Constitution on Divine Revelation,* section 9, in Flannery, *Vatican Council II.*

19. See John Paul II, *Christifideles Laici* (1989). The document is available on the Vatican website.

20. For an example of a call to the full Catholic community based on its commonly shared convictions and values that have been retrieved from the healing mission of Jesus, see Lloyd Dean and Deborah Proctor, "Honoring the Trust through Community Benefit," *Health Progress,* January-February 2007.

21. See Rodney Stark, *The Rise of Christianity: A Sociologist Reconsiders History* (Princeton: Princeton University Press, 1996), esp. chap. 4, "Epidemics, Networks, and Conversion."

22. For an understanding of continuity and change in Catholic traditions, see John E. Thiel, *Senses of Tradition: Continuity and Development in Catholic Faith* (New York: Oxford University Press, 2000). Chapter 3, "Dramatic Development as a Sense of Tradition," is especially pertinent to Catholic Health Care. It uses the example of the teaching on birth control as a possible candidate for dramatic development.

23. See Charles Bouchard, "Health Care as 'Ministry': Common Usage, Confused Theology," *Health Progress*, May-June, 2008.

24. Brian Yanofchick writes, "One of the more important and pleasant surprises of the committee's work was discovering real commonality in core content among existing formation programs. New circumstances and needs will always require constant re-evaluation of the content, and the depth may vary from system to system, but the following areas are represented in some way by all: Heritage, tradition and sponsorship, Mission and values, Vocation—call and response, Spirituality and theological reflection, Catholic Social Teaching, Ethics, Leadership

style, Holistic health care, Diversity, and Relationship to the broader church ministry." Yanofchick, "A Preview: CHA's Framework for Leadership Formation," *Health Progress,* September-October 2011. These general categories identify Catholic Health Care in this historical moment. However, for formation programming, what is important is the content of these categories and how this content is shaped as a leadership tool.

25. On the dialogic openness to the world that the Second Vatican Council recommends, see Richard McBrien, *The Church: The Evolution of Catholicism* (New York: HarperOne, 2008).

26. For example, in his encyclical *God Is Love*, Benedict XVI praises all the expanding forms of secular charity. But he traces their emergence and continuance to (1) the drive of God-given conscience for each person to love their neighbor and (2) the example of this type of charity that historical Christianity has provided. The community/tradition not only notes the positive movements of the larger culture. It also interprets them according to its own deepest convictions and values.

27. In Catholic theology, resistance is often associated with discerning the signs of the times. Discerning the signs of times entails conducting a social analysis in light of the Kingdom of God. What is happening in the world that is supporting God's call to a more unified humanity and what is happening in the world that undercuts that call? As history unfolds, it is necessary to evaluate this unfolding through the moral perspective that arises from a conscience that is grounded in God.

The reality of conscience and the need to continually allow it to influence perception and action is reaffirmed in the *Pastoral Constitution on the Church in the Modern World*: "Deep within his conscience man discovers a law which he has not laid upon himself but which he must obey. Its voice, ever calling him to love and to do what is good and to avoid evil, tells him inwardly at the right moment: do this, shun that. For man has in his heart a law inscribed by God. His dignity lies in observing this law and by it he will be judged. His conscience is man's most secret core, and his sanctuary. There he is alone with God whose voice echoes in his depths. By conscience, in a wonderful way, that law is made known which is fulfilled in the love of God and of one's neighbor." *Pastoral Constitution on the Church in the Modern World*, section 16, in Flannery, *Vatican Council II*. Both the law within the conscience of each individual and the Church's interpretation of that law ground the Catholic Health Care stance of resistance.

28. For the pervasiveness of secularity and the way it reshapes the options for religious sensibilities, see Charles Taylor, *A Secular Age* (Cambridge, Mass.: Belknap Press of Harvard University Press, 2007).

29. A mood is not so much one more philosophy as the background and foundation of all the philosophies and cultural creations of any given period. As a

constant and ever-present presupposition, mood enters into the shapes of consciousness, exerting tremendous influence on the character and scope of every undertaking. Langdon Gilkey identified "mood" as "that fundamental attitude toward reality, toward truth, and toward value which characterizes an epoch, and within whose terms every created aspect of life, including the period's religion and its theology, expresses itself." Gilkey, *Naming the Whirlwind* (Indianapolis: Bobbs-Merrill, 1969), 34. A similar evaluation of secularity is found in John Macquarrie, *God and Secularity* (Philadelphia: Westminster Press, 1967), 42–44.

30. For this reason secular humanism is often called exclusive humanism. See Charles Taylor, "A Catholic Modernity?" in *A Catholic Modernity?* ed. by James L. Heft (New York: Oxford University Press, 1999).

31. Paul VI pointed out this tension in the dialogue between the Church and the world: "The desire [for the Church and world] to come together must not lead to a watering-down or subtracting from the truth. Our dialogue must not weaken our attachment to our faith." It cannot lead us into "making vague compromises about the principles of faith and action." But, on the other hand, a person "must to a certain degree identify with the forms of life of those to whom he or she wishes to bring the message. . . . Without invoking privileges which would but widen the separation, without employing unintelligible terminology, he must share the common way of life—if he wishes to be listened to and understood" Paul VI, *Paths of the Church*, sections 88, 87. The translation of this encyclical is from the New Advent website.

Langdon Gilkey articulates this same balancing act: "The expression of the Gospel probably always requires that there be no total capitulation to any cultural *Geist*; and yet no formulation of the Gospel that is relevant or meaningful can possibly fail to express itself in categories familiar to its hearers." Gilkey, *Naming the Whirlwind*, 117.

32. "Integral Humanism" is a phrase associated with Jacques Maritain and his influential book *Humanisme Integral*, which, in its first translation into English, was titled *True Humanism*. But no matter what exact language is used, it is an idea that has wide appeal. Scattered throughout papal documents of the last fifty years are references to a "true" or "authentic" or "full" or "whole" humanism. From our perspective, these adjectives are meant to add the spiritual and corresponding ethical dimensions of the human to the secular emphasis. Therefore, they are part of a dialogue that recognizes the secular focus and then complements it with the content of Christian faith.

An example of integral humanism is John Paul II's assessment of development: "Development which is not only economic must be measured and oriented according to the reality and vocation of man seen in his totality, namely, according to his interior dimension. There is no doubt that he needs created goods and the products of industry, which is constantly being enriched by scientific and technological progress. And the ever greater availability of material goods not only meets needs but also opens new horizons. . . . However, in trying to achieve true development we must never lose sight of that dimension which is in the specific nature of man, who has been created by God in his image and likeness (cf. Gen 1:26)." John Paul II, *On Social Concern*, section 29. The translation comes from the Vatican website.

Benedict XVI positions "integral humanism" as the correction of a cultural bias toward relativism: "In the present social and cultural context, where there is a widespread tendency to relativize truth, practising charity in truth helps people to understand that adhering to the values of Christianity is not merely useful but essential for building a good society and for true integral human development." Benedict XVI, *Charity in Truth*, section 4. The translation is from the Vatican website.

Benedict XVI also sees "integral human development" as the inheritance of the Second Vatican Council and the driving force of the social teachings of Paul VI. These teachings communicated two important truths: "The first is *the whole Church, in all her being and acting—when she proclaims, when she celebrates, when she performs works of charity—is engaged in promoting integral human development. . . .* The second truth is that *authentic human development concerns the whole of the person in every single dimension.*" Ibid., section 11 (italics in original).

We think that this approach of integral humanism in the larger Catholic tradition can be brought into the formation efforts of Catholic Health Care with great benefit. It recognizes what a secular concentration has achieved as it criticizes and complements it.

33. The seven gifts of the Spirit are wisdom, understanding, counsel, fortitude, knowledge, piety, and fear of the Lord. The twelve fruits of the Spirit are charity, joy, peace, patience, kindness, goodness, long-suffering, humility, fidelity, modesty, continence, and chastity.

34. In the Catholic Health Association's Mission Centered Leadership Model, spiritual grounding is described as "the ability to reflect and call on the spiritual *resources* of the Catholic healthcare tradition, one's own personal faith, and the faith of one's coworkers. These personal and collective spiritual *resources* supply the deep grounding, motivation, and resolve that are necessary to carry out the ministry. They also provide the larger context of meaning for the day-in, day-out work of healthcare. The most effective Catholic healthcare leaders have an inner spiritual life that translates into external action."

This way of phrasing the concern of spirituality naturally connects it to ethics. Spirituality—the beliefs, stories, and practices that we use to become aware of and cooperate with the mysterious and ultimate Spirit that pervades our entire being, elevating, integrating, and transcending our physical and psycho-social nature—impels us to live in a loving way toward our neighbor.

35. Chapter 3, "Ministry Leadership Formation: Theological Grounding and Method," spells out this way of understanding theology.

36. "The question of God . . . must be posed as the question concerning the

supporting ground, the origin, and the future of the question that we ourselves are." Karl Rahner, *Theological Investigations* (New York: Crossroad, 1973), 9:139.

37. For the importance of getting the "right people" first, see Collins, *Good to Great*, chap. 3, "First Who . . . Then What."

38. After acknowledging that American workers are too diverse to discover what they "want" from work, James O'Toole and Edward E. Lawler III identify three needs that gainful employment satisfies: "(1) the need for basic economic resources and security essential to lead good lives; (2) the need to do meaningful work and the opportunity to grow and develop as a person; and (3) the need for supportive social relationships." O'Toole and Lawler, *The New American Workplace* (New York: Palgrave Macmillan, 2006), 8.

In a similar vein, Jeffrey Pfeffer enumerates four desires of American workers: "(1) interesting work that permits them to learn, develop, and have a sense of competence and mastery, (2) meaningful work that provides some feeling of purpose, (3) a sense of connection and positive social relations with their coworkers, and (4) the ability to live an integrated life, so that one's work role and other roles are not inherently in conflict and so that a person's work role does not conflict with his or her essential nature and who the person is as a human being." Pfeffer, "Business and the Spirit: Management Practices That Sustain Spirit," in *Handbook of Workplace Spirituality and Organizational Performance*, ed. Robert Giacalone and Carole L. Jurkiewicz (Armonk, N.Y.: M. E. Sharpe, 2003), 32.

For the challenge that workforce reduction brings to these desires of workers, see David Noer, *Healing the Wounds: Overcoming the Trauma of Layoff and Revitalizing Downsized Organizations* (San Francisco: Jossey-Bass, 2009). Workforce reduction challenges have a great impact on the immediate and long-range goals of formation.

CHAPTER 2

The Process and Content
of Leadership Formation

John Shea

Our formation praxis pushed us to articulate the meta-story of
Catholic Health Care as a changing community that carries a
founding revelation and creates developing traditions in interaction with a permeating culture. In a similar way, our praxis invited
us to develop a theory of how leaders could enter, participate
in, and be formed by this Catholic Health Care community and
tradition. In fact, with every decision we faced, the need for this
type of formation theory became more evident and more urgent.

Without theory, formation efforts are prone to become inconsistent and scattered. Many discordant pieces are brought forward
because each is individually appraised as important. But without
theory, it is difficult to decide how all these
important pieces can collaborate to produce
an integrated effect. With theory, programs
become more strategic. They know what to
include and what not to include, how to evaluate and how not to
evaluate, what to encourage and what not to encourage, what to
give credence to and what to ignore. Theory helps clarify goals
and implement strategies.

Theory helps clarify goals
and implement strategies.

However, even as we sought the benefits of theory, we were
aware of its limits, even dangers. Theory is often too neat, too

quick to package the diversity of experiences. Therefore, it will meet jarring, even contradictory, situations that challenge its assumptions. It will also encounter situations that fall completely outside its scope. If the theory is held too lightly, it may be flexible to the point of fickleness and too quickly abandoned. If the theory is held too tightly, it is tempting to overlook the jarring and ignore the new, even to resent them because they bring mess into an already constructed order. The middle position is to hold the theory firmly, accommodating new influences but not losing the foundation and direction it provides. We realize our theory must remain open, but we also realize it must retain the strengths of a theory.

Traditional Formation
and Leadership Formation

As we were piecing together a theory, we naturally drew on the perspectives and methods of traditional formation. Formation is a process that is referred to on every level of Catholicism, from episcopacy to parish. But our specific focus was on the entry and formation of women into the religious communities of their choice. Since it was women religious who founded, sustained, and developed our six systems, their formation was the predecessor experience and the obvious choice as the primary resource for leadership formation. In fact, some voices suggest that the formation path of women religious is normative. Its processes and procedures should be conserved and exported into leadership formation.[1] This would serve the agenda of continuity between the past and future. Connecting past and future leaders through a common formation experience would support the transition from sisters carrying the Catholic identity and mission to leaders carrying it. In fact, early in our program, leaders would often ask, "Is this the same formation that the sisters had?"

63

However, the participants in traditional formation and the participants in leadership formation have radically different life projects that unfold into different formation paths. The participants in traditional formation were women, usually young women, who were looking for a life calling in a community/tradition and a community/tradition that was looking for life-long committed members.[2] Formation was the path to discern an exclusive belonging to one another. Formation recognized stages (postulant, novice, levels of vows) and resulted in gradational forms of commitment to the community/tradition. In most cases, there was extensive formation and at least preliminary commitments before the women entered into ministries of their community/tradition. If they entered health care ministries, they applied to academic and professional programs in nursing, law, business, medicine, administration, and so on. They came to the work initially formed and committed to the work as a ministry of their community/tradition. But they had to acquire the credentials and skills that were needed to perform the ministry according to commonly agreed-upon standards. The sequence of this formation path was through formation that resulted in belonging to a community/tradition into the work of that community/tradition that required special education and training but was understood as a religiously motivated ministry.

> The participants in traditional formation and the participants in leadership formation have radically different life projects that unfold into different formation paths.

Leaders have different life projects and consequently different formation paths.[3] They are primarily people who have personal lives and are looking for the best possible work situation. They are dealing with the tensions and trade-offs of these two dimensions. As much as possible, they want the best compensation, the best work environment, and the most meaningful work. Most likely their work history has been a series of moves designed to integrate career ambitions and personal commitments. These moves have taken them into not-for-profit and for-profit, faith-based and non-faith-based health care. In the present work atmosphere, they are realistically ready for another move. They have the credentials and skills to do the work in their area of expertise and this makes them marketable in the health care world. But, at this moment, their organization has invited them into a formation experience that is designed to bring them into greater alignment with the Catholic identity and mission. The sequence of this formation path is through work understood as part of personal life into formation—at a certain point in their careers and at the request of the organization that presently employs them—to become more deeply aligned with the organizational mission, vision, and values that are informed and sponsored by a faith-based community/tradition.

Adoption and Adaption

This stark contrast between the situation of women religious and the situation of leaders has to be acknowledged and held steady. It makes any facile transfer of ideas or strategies from traditional formation to leadership formation suspect; and it keeps the focus on the real challenge. Leadership formation has to go through a process of adoption and adaption. Adoption recognizes the ancient wisdom of traditional formation and adaption recognizes the newness of the contemporary situation of leadership formation. The adoption-adaption process has to identify key perspectives and practices from traditional formation that are apt for organizational situations. Then, it has to shape those perspectives and practices so that they grow out of leadership responsibilities and are not perceived as ill-fitting impositions. Of course, the adoption-adaption process is in service of the formation goals—to develop the working knowledge and skills to lead the ministry and mission of Catholic Health Care.

We adopted and adapted four areas of traditional formation: (1) Traditional formation acknowledged the social fact of two involved parties—individuals and the community/tradition. We adapted this social fact to maintain a consistent focus on the relationship of the two involved parties—leaders and organization. (2) Traditional formation was triggered by a mutual interest between individuals and the community/tradition; and, as the formation process developed, the interest became a desire to become more connected to the community and to learn more about the tradition. We adapted this focus to determine leader interest at the beginning of the program and to create conditions throughout the program for the desire to belong to and continue the Catholic Health Care tradition. (3) Traditional formation unfolded by providing greater knowledge of the community/tradition and encouraging practices to internalize that knowledge. We adapted this combination of knowledge and practices into the organizational categories of the working knowledge and skills that leaders must have to lead the mission and ministry of Catholic Health Care and established a learning method that ensured that type of relevant knowledge and practical action. (4) Traditional formation believed that Spirit ultimately inspired the attraction and connection between individuals and a community/tradition. We adapted this sensitivity to spiritual agency and identified signs of its presence and inspiration in the creative, communal, and cumulative nature of the leadership formation process.

> Adoption recognizes the ancient wisdom of traditional formation and adaption recognizes the newness of the contemporary situation of leadership formation.

The significant cultural research around leadership development informed our adaption of traditional formation.[4] Since the basic formational change is from the world of religious communities into the world of organizational leadership, the more we know about that leadership world, the more effective the adaption will be. Leadership development identifies key areas of leadership, classifies competencies, and provides guidelines on how adult leaders learn in and through the challenges their situations present to them.

In short, it provides maps to the territories that the twelve foundational concerns want to influence. Although adaption highlights differences and insists they be respected, we found considerable overlap between the leadership formation agenda and leadership development research. In fact, some of this leadership development literature explicitly acknowledged spiritual traditions as part of its inspiration and direction or implicitly suggested agendas and exercises that have been the traditional territory of spiritual traditions.[5] Leadership formation and leadership development are natural partners in the project of excellence.[6]

Leaders and Organizational Culture

The first area of adoption-adaption maintains a sustained focus between the two involved parties—leaders and the organizational culture. This relationship is understood and accepted in the workplace. When people seek work and when organizations seek people to work, both make the distinction between technical and cultural fit. Technical fit has to do with the knowledge and skills that are needed for the position. Cultural fit involves alignment with the mission, vision, and values of the organization. Many job seekers and job interviewers think that determining technical fit is an easier task than determining cultural fit. Cultural fit is more intangible; but, in the long run, it often proves to be more important. Great skill that cannot fit eventually goes elsewhere, often leaving a good deal of consternation, if not devastation, in its wake—both for the ones who leave and the ones who remain.

> Our entire formation program lives in the relational space between leaders and organizational culture.

Our entire formation program lives in the relational space between leaders and organizational culture. To emphasize that space, we begin every session by framing it as an interaction between two involved parties. We ask the leaders to remember themselves as specialists. They have the credentials, experience, and expertise to be excellent at what they do. They are CEOs, COOs, CFOs, CMOs, and CNOs on system, regional, and local levels. A sampling of other titles would include chief quality officer, vice president of corporate responsibility, chief strategy officer, executive director of the foundation for international health, senior counsel, chief human resources officer, vice president of mission and chaplaincy, senior director of strategy and business development, vice president of corporate communications, chief information officer, chief strategy officer, executive director of physician services and development, vice president of construction, vice president of home care services, vice president of patient care services, and so on. Although the titles and combination of titles change from system to system, leaders from all the areas of contemporary health care participate in the formation program. Health care executives are gathered; and their individual work identities are acknowledged.

However, at this time in their work lives, they are exercising their expertise in the Catholic Health Care tradition. This tradition is embodied in each of their organizations; and MLC, in collaboration with these organizations, has identified twelve concerns of this tradition. These concerns constitute the organizational culture, and the reason these leaders are gathered is to gain greater alignment with this culture.[7] At lower levels of the organization, technical and cultural fits can be relatively separate. But once people move into managerial positions, the technical and cultural become more aligned; and when they become senior leaders, the technical and cultural are intimately related. The organizational culture and the organizational work mutually reinforce each other.

This is where formation happens. It is a systematic and sustained initiation into the Catholic culture of the organization. Of course, these leaders have known from the moment they applied and were hired that they were working for a Catholic operation.

In fact, many of them sought work in a Catholic organization precisely because of its faith-based grounding. Some have been to formation programs in the past; some have been in Catholic Health Care for a long time and have picked up the Catholic ethos through osmosis; some have only a minimal understanding of the Catholic tradition, basically what they heard at the orientation into the organization. Nevertheless, the invitation to be part of this program is seen as a step into a more advanced participation in the culture of the organization.

This advanced step is an appropriate requirement for a leadership position. Catholic Health Care is not easy to comprehend. It suffers from stereotypes, misinformation, and projections. Its complex reasoning is not expressed or communicated well. Most of all, its realistic yet hopeful appreciation of the mystery of people in community is not systematically elaborated and connected to the daily work of the organization. In short, Catholic Health Care has trouble telling its story to the very leaders who are carrying out its mission. If that is the case, then the ability of these leaders to tell the Catholic Health Care story to the organization as a whole and to the larger pluralistic culture is also compromised. Along with other purposes, leadership formation addresses this situation.

Determining Interest and Developing Desire

The second area of adoption-adaption builds on the first. In traditional formation, initial mutual interest between the involved parties was assumed. Individuals had enough interest to contact the community/tradition and inquire about the next steps to determine a possible match. The community/tradition was ready for this inquiry and had processes in place to engage the individuals. The two involved parties were mutually looking; and they found themselves looking at each other.

However, in organizational life the situation is quite different. The interest of the organization in the formation of leaders is shown by the very existence of a program. But the interest of leaders is an unknown quantity. The program is not mandatory; leaders are invited to participate. But everything in a deep-culture organization that comes from the top carries an implicit compliance message. The inner voice whispers: "If you do not accept the invitation, it might be a career-limiting decision." It is just not wise to refuse, even though there may be very little personal interest. Therefore, leadership formation has to inquire into interest and, once it is determined, it has to sustain interest throughout the formation process. Sustained interest unfolds into desire, and desire is essential for formation.

Unless leaders have an initial interest that eventually becomes a desire to belong to and continue the community/tradition of Catholic Health Care, they will not develop the discipline to learn the requisite working knowledge and skills. Therefore, at the first session of the program, we inquire into leaders' interest and give them the opportunity to articulate and assess their motivation for participating in formation. We ask leaders to share with one another: How were you asked to be part of this program? When you were asked, and what did you think about? Who did you talk to, and what did they say? Why did you say yes? Obviously, they have all said yes. But what is important for their participation in the program is the thought process that got them to yes. On the whole, they are very willing to share how they came to their decision and how they envision their participation.

> Unless individuals have an initial interest that eventually becomes a desire, they will not develop the discipline to learn the requisite working knowledge and skills.

It is impossible to communicate or even summarize all that is shared. But a double-sided observation is consistently made. According to the leaders, the organization is committed. On one side, it is committed to continuing its Catholic identity and mission into the future. Although many reasons are cited for this commitment, the clinching argument is simple. The organization is giving money, time, and personnel to a program in order to make this happen. On the other side, the organization is showing some commitment to the leaders themselves. It sees them as potentially a part of this Catholic Health Care future. Although their invitation does not protect them from downsizing or assure advancement, it is taken as a vote of confidence. They are on the organization's radar screen. Many feel honored to be asked and enter the program with good will, openness, interest, and readiness to cooperate. The underlying communication of a formation program is that the organization is committed to its Catholic identity and mission and is investing in leaders who can continue it.

A second exercise also deals with the question of interest. Leaders identify what they want to happen and what they don't want to happen in the program. There is always a strong consensus about what they don't want to happen—no proselytizing for the Catholic faith and no religious quarreling that will end up dividing them. Therefore, an important boundary is established. Belonging to the Catholic Health Care community/tradition does not entail any overt or covert evangelization. Of course, this boundary is fully shared by the organization and its tradition.

The consensus for what they want to happen can be put simply: they want the program to make a difference. They want to understand themselves and their work differently because of their participation in the program. Of course, at this point, the contours of this difference are not specifically spelled out. But, as we sometimes put it, they are eager for impact. They want to create a Catholic culture that will inform every aspect of the organization's activity. In the evaluation questions at the end of this session, we ask the leaders on a scale of one to ten, "Please rate your honest desire to participate in the next sessions of this program." This rating tells them and us if the basic condition of formation is in place: is there enough interest to begin? The numbers uniformly come back between eight and ten.

Perhaps the best inducement to interest and the development of desire is the essential partnership of the program. From the beginning the leaders have been co-designers with the MLC staff of what the program offers and how it is conducted. The major way this happens is through formal and informal evaluations. The experience of Group One changed the program for Group Two, the experiences of Groups One and Two changed the program for Group Three, and so on. Therefore, every new group has benefited from the groups who have gone before them; and groups who will come after them will benefit from their experience. At this point, four groups totaling around 500 leaders have completed the program and two groups totaling 240 leaders are presently in the program. We are approaching a critical mass in the six systems that has a cumulative effect on sustaining interest and developing desire.

This essential partnership extends into other areas. The MLC presenters and staff provide the working knowledge and skills of the twelve foundational concerns of Catholic Health Care. But the leaders themselves have to partner with us in two ways. First, we may present knowledge of the twelve concerns, but we do not know whether it is working knowledge. Does it connect with leadership activity? The leaders must evaluate the knowledge in light of its purpose and help us turn it into working knowledge. Second, although best practices are identified and shared, the program is not a set list of instructions about things to do. We have the agenda of articulation and integration of these concerns into organizational life. But only the leaders can decide how these concerns will work in their environment. Therefore, the program and leaders co-create each other. It is a partnership, a covenant, a dance in which both parties move together toward a common goal. This type of joint ownership builds interest and creates desire.

Knowledge and Practices

Traditional formation responded to interested individuals by providing them with knowledge of the community/tradition. If the interest was to unfold into desire and the desire was to eventuate in belonging to the community and continuing the tradition, greater knowledge was needed to facilitate that coming together. Accompanying this advance in understanding were practices. The practices (prayer, participation in the sacraments, spiritual direction, and so on) were geared to internalize the knowledge, to bring it beyond information into realization. The knowledge and the practices combined to form individuals into members of the community and advocates for the tradition.

We adopted this potent mix of knowledge and practices, but the adaption process entailed rigorous discernment around two questions. First, what is the requisite knowledge of the tradition? Even after the twelve foundational concerns have been identified, there is still a need to determine the specific content of these concerns. It has to be knowledge germane to Catholic Health Care and, more precisely, relevant to the responsibilities of leaders. Second, what are the practices that will internalize the knowledge? Practices included both the exercises that would be used to communicate the knowledge and the initiatives that leaders would take as a result of acquiring the knowledge. These two questions are at the heart of leadership formation.

Working Knowledge and Skills

The place to obtain knowledge of Catholic Health Care that is most familiar to leaders is the mission, vision, and values statements of their organizations.[8] These statements and other official documents are key formation texts. In particular, values have become important indicators of Catholic identity and mission. Some of the most mentioned values are respect, compassion, stewardship, justice, excellence, dignity, collaboration, and care for the poor.

These values are comparative, always reaching after better end-states. The organization is striving for greater justice, excellence, advocacy, and so on. But the values also point to a spirit in which everything is done. No matter the endeavor, it should be engaged in a spirit of respect, compassion, and so on. These values are not unique to Catholic Health Care. But, when they are taken together and integrated into a larger organizational picture, a distinctive way of being a contemporary health care organization emerges.

Identifying the Catholic Health Care organizational culture in the philosophical language of values connects it in a special way to Catholic social teaching. Catholic social teaching is addressed not only to Catholics but also to all people of good will. To talk to all people of good will, the teaching is often articulated in the philosophical language of principles and values. For example, it calls attention to the core principles and values of human dignity and the common good and the derived secondary principles and values that are addressed to particular situations—reverence for life, participation, subsidiarity, right of association, preferential option for the poor, and so on. In addition, since Catholic Health Care is directly concerned about the distribution of the medical goods of society and is itself a large-scale employer, it is called to exemplify Catholic social teaching as well as to be a player in bringing those teachings into the structuring of the larger society. Therefore, when Catholic Health Care names the community/tradition in terms of principles and values, it connects both to a commonly accepted cultural and organizational form and to Catholic social teaching.

When Catholic Health Care names the community/tradition in terms of principles and values, it connects both to a commonly accepted cultural and organizational form and to Catholic social teaching.

Espousing values and principles and driving them into policies and behaviors also clearly connects with leadership responsibility. Leaders are called to turn mission statements into tools of

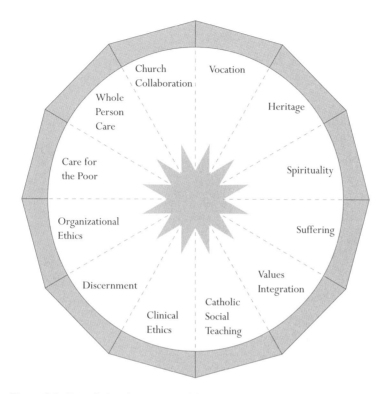

Figure 2.1 Foundational concerns of Catholic Health Care

organizational integrity. The stated values become assessment instruments to identify misalignments, create new alignments, and develop the ability to distinguish values from practices in order to lead change so that the larger purposes of the organization are not compromised. Values are also suitable for the condensed language of executive summaries and can be reliable touchstones for the many levels of decision-making that engage executives. So casting the knowledge of the Catholic Health Care tradition in terms of principles and values makes it user-friendly for leaders.

However, although values integration is a significant practice of Catholic Health Care, it cannot carry the whole agenda of the community/tradition. At MLC, we decided to include Values

Integration and Catholic Social Teaching as two of the concerns of the community/tradition. Then, through a process of inheritance, consultation, and intuition, we complemented them with ten other concerns—Vocation, Heritage, Spirituality, Responding to Suffering, Discernment, Whole Person Care, Care for the Poor, Organizational Ethics, Clinical Ethics, and Collaboration with Church Authorities and Agencies. (See figure 2.1.)

Deciding to present the tradition in the category of "concern" was a deliberate choice. There were other contenders—ingredients, aspects, features, facets, elements, areas of experience, and so on. But we settled on concern because it reinforced the essential partnership between MLC and the leaders of the six systems. The concerns are established, but how leaders would implement them was the work of creative connection. To emphasize this leadership responsibility, we transposed the twelve concerns into an avowal statement of the identity and work of leaders in Catholic Health Care. The first year focused on the identity:

> As leaders in Catholic Health Care, we understand ourselves as (1) called to this work (2) in the context of a ministerial tradition that ultimately takes its inspiration and direction from the healing mission of Jesus. As part of this tradition, (3) we are committed personally and professionally to the spiritually grounded values (4) that guide our work in responding to human suffering.

The second and third years focus on the work:

> As leaders in Catholic Health Care, we work (5) to integrate core values into organizational structures, policies, and behaviors; (6) to link discernment to strategic decision-making, innovation, and team composition; (7) to incorporate the Catholic social tradition into organizational life and mission; (8) to develop and ensure accountability for ethical policies, practices, and behaviors in our clinical settings; (9) to develop and ensure accountability for ethical policies, practices, and behaviors in our organizational relationships;

(10) to bring the benefits of healthcare to the poorest and most vulnerable members of our society; (11) to respect and attend to the whole person of patients, physicians, associates, and volunteers; (12) to work collaboratively with Church authorities and agencies.

We characterize the requisite knowledge of each of these twelve concerns as working. This type of knowledge is meant to be an alternative to two other possibilities. The first is knowledge for its own sake. These twelve concerns could be explored biblically, theologically, ethically, historically, and organizationally. There is no shortage of material. But this comprehensive approach has to be disciplined, and material has to be selected that ties into health care in general and leadership in particular. The second is knowledge as a data dump. Although basic information is always needed, it has to be accompanied by context and purpose for it to have formation potential. Knowledge characterized as working avoids knowledge for its own sake and knowledge that is merely an accumulation of ideas and positions. Working knowledge is the meeting place of MLC and the leaders. It brings together MLC's value of relevance, which creatively links our work to the lived experience of participants, and the request of the participants that they be given something that makes a difference. Working knowledge connects these two agendas.

To emphasize this leadership responsibility, we transposed the twelve concerns into an avowal statement of the identity and work of leaders in Catholic Health Care.

However, this emphasis on working knowledge cannot lead to a narrow focus on practicality. The administrative mind values execution and so tips for getting things done are eagerly received, judiciously evaluated, and quickly adapted to diverse circumstances. Of the three questions "why," "what," and "how," "what" is being done and "how" it is being done are the default comfort zones of leaders. But formation also embraces the "why" question, bringing into work situations the organizational rationale for what is being done and the motivation of individuals to enthusiastically join the effort. Working knowledge covers the whole spectrum of the human person.

This fuller understanding of relevance led us from discriminating what possibly might be working knowledge to observing how the knowledge of the twelve concerns was actually working. What was it doing for the leaders? We observed the knowledge working in four different ways—application, theory, interiority, and transcendence.[9] It was working in an application mode when it could be transferred directly into a work situation. It was working in a theoretical mode when it provided deeper reasons and critical focus. It was working in an interior mode when it addressed self-understanding and attitudes. Finally, it was working in a transcendent mode when it provided big picture perspectives and inspiration. In all these ways, it was relevant to both the personal and professional life of leaders.

As leaders grasp the knowledge that is distinctive to Catholic Health Care and become comfortable in the ways that knowledge works, they develop their own voice.

There are two skills that accompany the working knowledge of the twelve concerns—articulation and integration. These practices bring greater internalization of the knowledge and at the same time put the knowledge in service of organizational identity and mission. These two skills are connected to the program locations—off-site and on-site. "Off-site" refers to the leaders gathered together at a retreat house for a day-and-a-half session on one of the twelve concerns. "On-site" is when they return to their workplaces with plans on how to use what they have learned. Articulation begins off-site and continues on-site; integration is planned off-site and executed on-site.

As leaders grasp the knowledge that is distinctive to Catholic Health Care and become comfortable in the ways that knowledge works, they develop their own voice. They find ways to articulate the dynamics of the twelve concerns. This voice truly differs from person to person, but there are two qualities that are usually developed across the diversity. The leader's voice is initiatory. For the most part, co-workers and publics are not going to ask for the Catholic ethos to enter the conversation. The leader is going to have to bring it in, volunteer it amid business talk. This means that the voice must also be strategic. It must assess situations in terms of opportunities, take into account the receptivity of co-conversationalists, and determine the added value of explicitly bringing the Catholic identity and mission to bear on the matter at hand. Initiation and strategy guide the development of the skill of articulation.

This ability to articulate develops in tandem with integration. It is important that integration is truly integration and not accumulation, one more thing to do. As leaders look at their calendar of upcoming activities, they need to determine which of those activities would be enhanced by bringing forward some of the working knowledge they have learned. This is a skill that has a wide range of development. At first there does not seem to be any opportunity and eventually there seem to be many. The leaders find ways to bring what they are learning into their work situations. In this way, they strengthen the culture of the organization and mark it as distinctively Catholic. They gradually become both confident and competent in articulating and integrating the Catholic identity and mission.

Learning Method

How the twelve foundational concerns are learned has to serve the goals of providing working knowledge and skills. Learning method and learning goals have to be aligned. We adopted, experimented with, and tailored a pastoral model known as the Triangle.[10] The three points of the Triangle are Catholic tradition, cultural information, and individual and communal experience. (See figure 2.2.) The Catholic tradition sets the agenda. It names the twelve concerns and positions each in the middle of the Triangle. In addition to identifying the concerns, the Catholic tradition provides theological perspectives about why these concerns are important, ethical guidelines for addressing them, and insights into their implications. Cultural information informs the agenda. It includes pertinent data from the social sciences, cultural analyses, contemporary philosophies, and, most of all, current organizational protocols and processes. Finally, individual and communal experience evaluates the concerns. The leaders use past experience to assess the material from the Catholic tradition and the cultural information and determine what they want their future experience to be.

This learning method is an apt model for developing the working knowledge and skills of the twelve concerns. The tradition identifies the areas of knowledge that make up the mission and ministry. But it immediately combines those areas with current cultural assumptions and information and, in the process, makes that knowledge "working" and relevant to the organizational challenges of health care. Then as the tradition and culture come together into working knowledge, they consult the experience of the leaders. The leaders articulate how this working knowledge relates to their situations and how it can be integrated into the organizational life and mission. The three points of the Triangle are in ongoing interaction with one another, contributing to the development of working knowledge and skills.

This learning method has two additional benefits. Leaders appropriate it as a checklist for other situations. Whatever they are attending to is put into the center of the Triangle. Then, as the conversation and decision-making develop, they make sure the tradition is represented, the culture is considered, and the experience of the multiple stakeholders is taken into account.[11] There is also a programmatic advantage to this learning method. It supplies

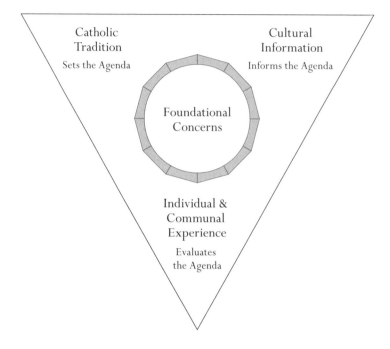

Figure 2.2 Learning model of the Ministry Leadership Formation Program

unity to a program that is long on diversity. Over a three-year period, twelve different concerns are considered. Without some form of unity, something that consistently holds the twelve together, the program would appear a laundry list, piecemeal and scattered. When the same learning method is applied to each concern, it provides a uniform procedure that gives order and direction to the whole.

Creative, Communal, and Cumulative

Traditional formation believed that spiritual influences assisted the growing relationship between individuals and the community/tradition. These influences were invisible and hidden, but they were also operative within the more available psychological states and social dynamics. Although they could not be directly accessed, their effects could be observed. In particular, if certain things were happening—like greater peace, happiness, energy toward mission, and so on—it was assumed that the relationship between individuals and the community/tradition was being supported and directed by spiritual energies.

This was a subtle discernment. The individuals and the community/tradition brought good will, knowledge, and practices to each other and engaged the process with integrity. But as they interacted, something would or would not occur that they recognized was beyond their control. They could create conditions for this something to happen, but they could not make that something happen. Therefore, when it did occur, they acknowledged that another agency was involved. The Spirit who has the reputation of making all things one was bringing the individuals and the community/tradition together for their own good and the good of others.

Traditional formation displayed a generosity toward human complexity. Leadership formation should do no less.

Of course, the development of a symbiosis between individuals and the community/tradition was not the only outcome of formation processes. Individuals and the community/tradition split, or they connected with each other for a short period of time and then they went their separate ways, or a good relationship soured, or an initial match continued to deepen and full humanity flowered, or individuals heard other calls, or other countless scenarios. But no matter what happened, the sine qua non of the process was the assumption that a deeper Spirit was at work. As long as discernment of this Spirit was present, the outcomes were evaluated as providentially guided. Paradoxically, formation made possible belonging to the community and continuing the tradition, but it also brought clarity to matches that were not working and an encouragement to find other paths. Traditional formation displayed a generosity toward human complexity. Leadership formation should do no less.

Despite its significant differences from traditional formation, leadership formation should take into account this combination of human effort and spiritual influence. This is partly because of the centrality of this belief and its practice in Catholic Christianity. Not to honor it would be more than an oversight. It might signal an undue capitulation to the restrictions of secular consciousness. The business world may look askance at this way of thinking and acting, and the drive to have credibility in that world might seduce us into uncritically conforming to those confinements. This is a typical way important pieces of the tradition are lost. They are not refuted; they just make people uncomfortable.

But an equally important reason for holding together human effort and spiritual influence is that it seems to fit the actual experience of leadership formation. As the process unfolds, some leaders find a home and others come to realize they might be in the wrong place. Some grow on professional and personal levels; others are basically unaffected. Ones who protest at first praise at last; and ones who praise at first languish at last. There is a mystery of attraction and growth going on beneath the dogged efforts to provide the working knowledge and skills necessary to lead the mission and ministry of Catholic Health Care. It is as old as the spiritual adage: man proposes, but God disposes.

MLC and the leaders, in essential partnership, do everything they can for formation to be successful. Then something happens or it does not. When it happens, formation becomes creative, communal, and cumulative.

This spiritual assumption translates into a formation strategy. At MLC, we put in place the best ways of educating adults in organizational settings. We hone the concerns of the tradition until they yield working knowledge and we sharpen the skills of articulation and integration until they are ready to flow easily and naturally into leadership situations. In short, MLC and the leaders, in essential partnership with each other, do everything they can for formation to be successful. And then something happens or it does not. When it happens, it is easily identified. The formation process becomes creative, communal, and cumulative.

The formation process is creative when it holds together the personal and the professional sides of the leader. When leaders see their personal selves in the concerns of the tradition, they begin establishing strong ties to the organizational culture. For example, in the Vocation session, leaders often comment that their work has always had a vocational character, but that they never gave it credence until they saw how important it was to the organization. Or, from the Responding to Suffering session, leaders return home to sick family members or neighbors with a desire to be present to them. In short, through their formation they are becoming, by their own estimate, fuller and better people. This is perhaps the highest compliment a formation program can receive.

This connection to the person of the leader is paralleled by a connection to the profession of the leader. Most leaders strive for excellence. The very fact they have advanced into leadership positions witnesses to that. When their formation process shows them paths of excellence they had not previously seen, they are inspired to perform in new ways and they establish deeper connections to the organizational culture. For example, in the Discernment session, leaders discover inner disciplines that are helpful to effective decision-making. Or, in the Organizational Ethics session, they assess and improve their present way of communicating decisions that were the result of ethical struggles. In fact, all the sessions are designed to have maximum professional impact. When they do, leaders move into wholeness, integrating both the personal and professional into their role.

However, the relationship between leaders and the organizational culture will always be a mixed bag. Although leaders grow into greater conformity with the organizational culture, there will always be disagreement and tension. The leader is never absorbed into the organization, and the organization is never collapsed into the leader. Leaders may resonate with some aspects of the organizational culture and respect other aspects, even though they do not resonate with them. But there will always be aspects leaders want reviewed and changed. Creativity is forging connections that are capacious enough to house disconnections and recognizing that belonging includes criticism, even welcomes it.

Creativity develops within community. The formation process is communal because by its very nature it situates the individual leaders within collective conversations. Its natural environment is overlapping communities. It includes people at home and people at work, people who have been through previous formation cohorts, people who compose the staff of MLC, and people who present at each session. In short, anyone who enters into the formation conversation with leaders becomes part of the communal context of their development.

However, pride of place belongs to the members of the formation cohort (the forty leaders who go through the three-year program together). These conversations, both in formal sessions and over drinks and meals, informed and sharpened the formation process. When the initial program concludes and invitations are sent out for further sessions, the primary reason leaders come is to see the people who shared their formation. Catholic social teaching insists we are social by nature, and we remind ourselves of this truth with the phrase "we are better together than we are alone." When we experience this enhanced self within a certain community, we want to rejoin that community whenever we are able.

However, the communal process is not in the sheer fact of individual and community interaction. It is in how community develops in relation to mission. The classic question is, does the community have a mission or does the mission have a community? If like-minded people come together and establish ties with one another and then decide on some communal action, then a community has a mission. If people come together around a mission, a task they are all committed to, and in the process form communal ties in order to do the task more effectively, the mission has a community. In leadership formation, the mission has a community. As people share their organizational situations and their leadership challenges, they find a degree of support that turns the formation process communal.

The creativity that happens within community is cumulative. In formation, the emphasis is on personal consciousness change and the behaviors that will emerge from the change. This consciousness change can be expected, but it cannot be predicted; and it definitively cannot be forced. But it does presuppose a beginning, a moment of awakening. It may be too dramatic to call this moment a breakthrough. But after it happens, consciousness grows and behaviors develop faster. A common refrain of leaders is: "It was around the fifth session [out of twelve] that I got it." A learning process was always at work, but the awakening came in the fifth session.

The awakening triggers cumulative development in earnest. Intellectual integration begins to happen—seemingly on its own. Ideas previously known fall into place and new knowledge fits into this growing gestalt. This mental activity is the precursor to behavioral change; and it is developing because of its exposure to and internalization of the working knowledge of the twelve foundational concerns. In the parable language of the Gospels, the word has found good soil.

> As people share their organizational situations and their leadership challenges, they find a degree of support that turns the formation process communal.

Once awakening happens, cumulative development continues as an unfolding of knowledge. The mapped stages of this unfolding are from information to understanding, from understanding to realization, and from realization to integration.

Knowledge arrives as information. For example, Catholic Health Care emphasizes care for the poor. This knowledge may advance into understanding—Catholic Health Care emphasizes care for the poor because its conviction of the spiritual unity of the human race critiques the great discrepancy in the distribution of the goods of the earth. This understanding may advance into realization when it moves from what the organizational culture holds to what leaders, both personally and professionally, embrace. Finally, realization

The awakening triggers cumulative development in earnest. Ideas previously known fall into place and new knowledge fits into this growing gestalt.

advances into integration when leaders find ways to bring their transformed consciousness into their leadership activities.

When formation is happening, the working knowledge of the twelve foundational concerns is being appropriated and the skills of articulating and integrating these concerns are being developed. This actualized potential is manifested in the creative, communal, and cumulative quality of the development. MLC and the leaders have put their hand to the plough to make this formation happen. They created the conditions for the possibility of this to happen. Yet when it does happen, it seems to come as a gift. Something more is at work. It is only right to acknowledge Spirit.

Conclusion

Throughout its long history, Catholic Health Care has been a changing community that has carried a founding revelation and has created developing traditions in response to a permeating culture. The contemporary interaction of these meta-story components— community, revelation, tradition, and culture—is the context for formation initiatives. The changing community takes the form of a complex and stratified work organization. This organization is inviting its leaders into a deeper relationship with the foundational concerns of its tradition. With this invitation, both the organization and the leaders have decisions and responsibilities. The organization has to clearly identify the working knowledge of its foundational concerns and provide structural and attitudinal support for leaders to develop the ability to articulate and integrate these concerns. The leaders, in turn, have to discern their initial interest, cultivate an ever-deepening desire, and engage the working knowledge and develop the skills to continue the tradition. This teamwork of organization and leaders is the constitutive element of the formation experience. On a deep level, both the organization and the leaders should be aware that a creative, communal, and cumulative process of belonging and meaning is unfolding.

Notes

1. Doing formation within organizational life is a new location. Formation ideas and strategies that were developed in novitiates and seminaries cannot be exported whole cloth. In those settings, the formation tools of scripture and liturgy were used in a certain way, prayer and reflection went on in a certain way, and ethical behavior was encouraged and critiqued in a certain way. None of these ways fit well into organizational life. Attempts to make them fit have proved awkward and, quite literally, out of place.

2. In this context, "community/tradition" does not refer to the community/tradition of Catholic Health Care. It refers to the community/tradition of the religious order, one of whose ministries is health care.

3. Early in the program, many of leaders, both men and women, would ask, only half in jest, "Are you going to try and make me into a nun?"

4. For the close and complementary connections between leadership development and leadership formation, see John O. Mudd, "When Knowledge and Skills Aren't Enough," *Health Progress*, September-October 2009.

5. See, among others, Mark Gerzon, *Leading through Conflict* (Cambridge, Mass.: Harvard Business School Press, 2006); Robert A. Giacalone and Carole L. Jurkiewicz, *Handbook of Workplace Spirituality and Organizational Performance* (Armonk, N.Y.: M. E. Sharpe, 2003); Daniel Goleman "What Makes a Leader?" *Harvard Business Review*, November-December 1998; Peter Senge, *The Fifth Discipline* (New York: Doubleday, 1990); Kerry A. Bunker, Douglas T. Hall, Kathy E. Kram, eds.,

Extraordinary Leadership: Addressing the Gaps in Senior Executive Development (San Francisco: Jossey-Bass, The Center for Creative Leadership, 2010); Richard Boyatzis and Annie McKee, *Resonant Leadership* (Cambridge, Mass.: Harvard Business School Press, 2005).

6. Chapter 4, "The Relationship between Leadership Development and Leadership Formation," spells out this partnership in detail.

7. For the importance of leaders shaping the organizational culture in a desired direction, see Terrence F. Deal and Allan A. Kennedy, *Corporate Cultures* (Boston: Addison-Wesley, 1982); and Edgar H. Schein, *Organizational Culture and Leadership* (San Francisco: Jossey-Bass, 1992).

8. Of course, knowledge of Catholic Health Care can be obtained from the *Ethical and Religious Directives* of the National Conference of Catholic Bishops and from the many publications and the website of the Catholic Health Association. But the most available source is what is closest.

9. We are grateful to John Fontana for suggesting these categories. When we used them, they fit to a remarkable degree.

10. James D. Whitehead and Evelyn Eaton Whitehead introduced the Triangle into pastoral theology in *Method in Ministry: Theological Reflection and Christian Ministry* (New York: Seabury Press, 1980).

11. Chapter 3, "Ministry Leadership Formation: Theological Grounding and Method," elaborates on the dialogic interaction of the three points of the Triangle.

CHAPTER 3

Ministry Leadership Formation Theological Grounding and Method

Laurence J. O'Connell

Ministry leadership formation requires a distinctive approach to incorporating theological content and perspective. This distinctive theological style flows naturally from the dynamic, cumulative nature of the formation process and its primary objective, namely, personal transformation in service of organizational transformation. The constant back and forth of the formation experience calls for a personal, conversational tack that emphasizes informative dialogue and emergent self-reflection rather than theoretical precision. An overly formal, academic approach to the theological foundations of ministry leadership runs the risk of providing abstract theory without sufficiently integrating concrete, practical leadership problems and issues. The desired transformative effect of formation could be muffled by an undue preoccupation with theological concepts and their manipulation. Make no mistake, though: an underlying theological foundation must be firmly in place. Bringing it forth and integrating it with the experience of the participants requires a process of personal appropriation rather than pedantic rigor on the part of facilitators.

As we shall see, the substantive role of theology lies at the heart of the formation process. Yet questions of style are also important. Given the formidable life experience and the diversity among our participants—for example, age, ethnicity, gender, race, sexual orientation, and religious affiliation—we intentionally make our approach invitational and encompass it in an adult education design that builds on the sustained attention to the experience of the participants and the sustained theological presence of the experienced formational guides.

Invitational Design

We are convinced that the theological component of ministry formation for adult lay leaders in today's health care environment must be invitational as leaders enter the formation experience with varied theological understandings. The approach must be unambiguously distanced from any hint of coercive intent.

In our first session, we emphatically state that our invitation to theological reflection is not a disguised attempt to lure unwitting executives into the ranks of institutional Catholicism. We are not hawking the Catholic tradition. Sometimes we are greeted with laughter; but we have also heard more than one sigh of relief! On the contrary, our approach is an explicit attempt to honor what Pope Paul VI called "the duty of welcoming others."[1] And we accept Pope Benedict XVI's caution against "engaging in what is nowadays considered proselytism" and his reminder that "those who practice in the Church's name must never seek to impose the Church's faith upon others."[2]

> Our bottom-up approach uses existing participant experience as an entry point for bridging theological concepts with the concrete events, relationships, and circumstances that define their real-life world.

In line with a welcoming posture, we believe that theological perspective is best understood and appreciated when it rises from below, from the lived experience of participants, meeting them where they are. We explicitly acknowledge the value of their own personal experience and spiritual point of view. As Pope Paul VI insisted:

a person must to a certain degree identify with the forms of life of those to whom he or she wishes to bring the message. . . . Without seeking privileges which would but widen the separation, without employing unintelligible terminology, he or she must share the common way of life . . . if he or she wishes to be listened to and understood.[3]

As participants encounter the Catholic tradition at close range, they are encouraged to compare their own values and personal attitudes and religious (or non-religious) experiences with the core concerns of Catholic social thought and imagination. We encourage them to seek out and, wherever possible, reinforce relevant lines of connection with their personal spiritual understanding and traditions as they test for overall compatibility between the Catholic tradition and their own angle of moral vision and behavior.

To enhance accessibility, we underscore our belief that the Roman Catholic tradition has a message and is called to a mission that resonates with the heartfelt longings and moral aspirations of all people of good will. One may not agree with certain particulars, but core concerns like justice, human dignity, and the common good do elicit a sympathetic hearing from most people. Picking up on the thinking of John Paul II, we consider ourselves "a partner in humanity's shared struggle to arrive at the truth."[4]

> To enhance accessibility, we underscore our belief that the Roman Catholic tradition has a message and a mission that resonates with the heartfelt longings and moral aspirations of all people of good will.

Our theological path is patterned on those who seek a via media, a middle way that is steadfastly committed to the core teachings of the Catholic tradition but that embraces dialogue with the world's religious and spiritual traditions. In principle, we steer clear of ideological extremes. On the one hand, we avoid the conceited absolutism that adopts a standpoint of exclusivity (where other perspectives are simply ruled out of court) and superiority (where Roman Catholicism is seen as a priori better in doctrine, ethics, or system). On the other hand, we expressly disavow irresponsible relativism. We are firmly in the camp of those who "consider an arbitrary pluralism untenable, the view that approves and endorses without differentiation both one's own and the other religions, without calling attention to the presence in both groups of untruth despite all the truth."[5]

Our executive leaders find a source of encouragement in our companionable approach. They report a sense of freedom to be themselves in reflection and dialogue. Participants begin to relax and trust one another, thereby setting the stage for ongoing theological reflection that values the insights of the Catholic tradition while welcoming interfaith and ecumenical perspective.

The whole process unfolds within a spirit of reciprocal respect. Participants begin to lean into the tradition and understand how they can authentically assimilate its core theological values. The result is a definite sense of identification and ownership with core concepts. Empirical evaluation has demonstrated that the invitation to explore and personally connect with the theological foundations of the tradition leads to a solid sense of belonging to a rich and truly human organizational culture, whether or not someone is Catholic.[6]

Theology makes its way into executive practice over time through a type of osmosis that respects personal integrity yet honestly and unapologetically stimulates reflection through a Catholic worldview. As in osmosis, there is an identifiable but permeable separation that allows for mutuality and life-giving transference. Although complete identification with the theological tradition is not expected of all participants, a high degree moral congruence is essential. A Muslim chief executive officer, for instance, need not believe in the divinity of Jesus Christ; but she is unquestionably bound to manage operations in a manner consistent with basic Catholic values and the Catholic moral vision.

Still even our invitational style poses a number of challenges for the facilitators who guide the formation process while sensitively attending to spiritual and theological dimensions. We have adopted an approach that we hope is artful yet substantive and credible as well as pedagogically suitable and theologically solid.

Adult Orientation

In our effort to meet the participants on their own ground, we draw upon the principles of adult learning that place a premium on collaboration and mutual respect. Adults expect to be consulted about the agenda, underlying assumptions, and expected outcomes. They appreciate a conversational style marked by intimacy, interactivity, inclusion, and intentionality.[7] When they feel patronized or manipulated, executive leaders simply check out, and any attempt to address sensitive value-based questions and theological concerns is undercut.

We have also learned that practical and problem-centered examples are most effective in eliciting a rich dialogue around deeply personal yet professionally relevant topics. For example, we juxtapose the theological notion of vocation with current trends in business practice. Today's business literature distinguishes between job, career, and calling. We ask, how does this distinction relate to the theological idea of vocation and how might it influence your leadership in a faith-based organization? In this way, we respond to the requirements of adult learners who expect their formation experience to be grounded in and oriented toward practice, and who appreciate the opportunity to apply the formation experience to their actual work experience. Any failure to meet their reasonable expectation to include their personal leadership experience diminishes their willingness to invest in the formation process. Indeed, such a failure may unwittingly foreclose opportunities to get to where the spiritual and theological wellsprings of personal transformation reside.

Experienced Formational Guides

While the pedagogical approach to the theological dimensions of ministry leadership formation is critical, the background and ability of those entrusted with guiding the process are no less important. Facilitators must have a firm grasp of the Catholic tradition, its historical development, and issues affecting Catholic Health Care and be experienced in guiding theological reflection in this context.

As already noted, the invitational and dialogical method places some exceptional demands on the theologians guiding the formation process. For example, they are not afforded the luxury of preparing carefully crafted presentations, so they must be quick on their feet and capable of engaging in rapid-fire dialogue, but they must remain surefooted in safeguarding doctrinal integrity and clarity. They must avoid the easy out of offering up simplistic formulas or pat answers. Moreover, they must be prepared to use the emergent issue at hand to retrieve and relate theological themes that appeared earlier in the program, constantly weaving a consistent pattern as the theological cloth of the formation process is spun out over three years.

> This balanced amalgam of receptive participant, trusted guide, and respectful process inspires confidence, invites sharing, and opens the inner space where the real work of formation takes place.

We have found that an invitational style coupled with adult learning skills and experienced guides reduces mental and emotional resistance to communicating personally and transparently, the sine qua non of effective theologically grounded formation. This balance of receptive participant, trusted guide, and respectful process inspires confidence, invites sharing, and opens the inner space where the real work of formation takes place. The fact that this inner space is continually crisscrossed with spiritual and theological concerns ultimately draws little attention; since suspicions of ulterior motives have earlier been debunked, participants have come to trust the competent guidance of the facilitators, and they are now confident that the work is grounded in and oriented toward practice.

This careful positioning allows the move into the substance of theology and its impact on leadership in Catholic Health Care organizations to be far less complicated than one might think. Clearing the way is very important. Although ministry leadership formation is not about teaching theology per se, it is profoundly theological.

Dialogical Method: The Triangle

In chapter 2, we introduced our learning method and gave an overview of the Triangle, which serves as the paradigm. In this section, we will explore the theological dimension of the model and more explicitly align it with the distinctive Catholic approach to tackling contemporary issues as they arise and influence various areas of practice, for example, health care. As we shall see, the Triangle is a perennial feature, a constant within the Catholic Christian tradition.[8] In 1980, James and Evelyn Whitehead applied this age-old approach in articulating a systematic way to mine the various sources of religious information in a manner that would lead beyond theoretical insight to actual decisions. In their model, three sources of insight—the Christian tradition, cultural perspectives, and personal experience—are juxtaposed and placed into critical dialogue. The mutual interaction of the three sources generates fresh theological perspectives that open the way for timely yet theologically informed responses to contemporary circumstances. (See figure 3.1.)

Influenced by major developments in the field of practical theology, the Whiteheads in 1995 substantially revised the original edition, which had been published in 1980.[9] In 2005, the Ministry

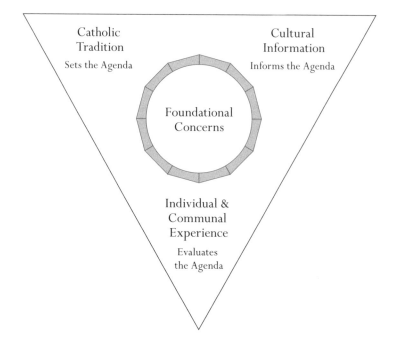

Figure 3.1 Learning model of the Ministry Leadership Formation Program

Leadership Center adopted and over time refined the Triangle to our own self-understanding and purposes. In retrospect, our choice was providential. The Triangle has become a central unifying feature in the work of expanding knowledge, honing skills, and shaping the attitudes of health care leaders in ten western States. Our participants report that the Triangle is now routinely deployed in discernment processes as well as in discussions of moral priorities, strategic direction, and tactical preferences. Thus, the Triangle serves as an icon, providing a shared vocabulary, moral compass, and methodological structure during and after the completion of the three-year formation experience.

The Triangle is a deceptively simple but very efficient way to describe what one might call the survival strategy of the Roman

Catholic tradition. It is shorthand for the process of theological reflection that serves as the living link between the past and the present. It ensures that "the appeal to tradition is not mere remembrance of the past," but a call "to develop for the future an original, new, and constructive mode of thinking." [10]

Our participants report that the Triangle is now routinely deployed in discernment processes as well as discussions of moral priorities, strategic direction, and tactical preferences.

The three points of the Triangle represent intersecting sources, forces, or repositories of relevant insight and information. Each source— that is, religious heritage, contemporary culture, and personal and communal experience—is indispensable. The tradition depends on spirited, critical exchange between these three sources for its very survival. Although Jan Walgrave never encountered the Triangle as we know it, he was certainly in touch with the tradition's drive for survival through self-renewal and adaptation:

> It [tradition] always tries to fit the expression of faith into patterns of contemporary thought. . . . Its attitude toward contemporary thought is at once assimilative and critical. It is always in the process of creating, retouching, and correcting a system of thought in which the equilibrium between revelation and the modern mind is maintained and constantly restored through an interchange that is at once a dialogue and a conflict. [11]

The dialogical interplay of the past and present opens a path to the future that, as Pope John XXIII insisted, is designed "to meet the needs of our time." The Triangle is not a pedagogical novelty; it is the contemporary expression of perennial practice.

The relevance of this approach to contemporary ministry formation and its significance for anyone who is charged with leading a Catholic Health Care organization in the twenty-first century are unquestionable. In outlining the many forces that threaten Catholic Health Care's future, William J. Cox underscored the need to deploy the assimilative power of Catholicism's method of theological triangulation. In discussing the contention that the dissipation of the Catholic mission in institutional health care is well under way, Cox maintained that we need "to find ways and means of renewing the religious character of our health care institutions and enabling the next generation of leaders to both own it and transmit it. . . . Our responsibility is to retrieve and nurture that legacy in our institutions and pass it on in its fullness to the next generation."[12]

The Ministry Leadership Center's approach to theological reflection represents a response to this insightful call. It is the Center's mission to conserve, explicate, and transmit Catholicism's rich heritage to those who are entrusted with the Church's health care ministries. In other words, the Center serves as a living link between the teachings of the Catholic Christian tradition and a world of culture in continuous development. As such, the Center is part of the theological enterprise itself, seeking to honor the tradition while both respecting and challenging culture in ways that resonate with the individual and communal experiences of our participants. The Center provides space and time for a style of spiritual and theological reflection that is deeply embedded in the Catholic approach to bringing the interests of the tradition to bear on ever-changing circumstances over time. Our understanding of the Triangle, that is, as representing the dynamic movement of the Catholic tradition, informs our choices and guides our work.

We have fashioned our approach to the Triangle along lines that allow it to function as an overarching framework that provides easy access to the workings of the Catholic tradition (its *descriptive function*), and as a template for leadership behavior (its *existential function*). Although understanding its descriptive function plays an important role in developing knowledge and skills, it is the Triangle's existential function that shapes fundamental attitudes that in turn induce the transformative effects of formation. On the descriptive level, the Triangle is a learning method and serves an instrumental purpose. It is useful. On the existential level, the Triangle serves a theological purpose. It is personal and thus inherently meaningful.

The distinction between the descriptive and existential functions of the Triangle is important. On the descriptive level, the Triangle is an object to be manipulated. On the existential level, the Triangle is a way of life to be appropriated and enacted. Both functions have their proper place and legitimate role. They work in tandem to inform and propel the formation process, fueling the twin engines of articulation and integration.

> Grasping the existential and theological purpose of the Triangle is an eye opener for our participants. They begin to understand themselves as agents of the tradition, stewards of the living, dynamic, and cumulative heritage entrusted to them.

Grasping the existential, indeed theological, purpose of the Triangle is an eye opener for our participants. They wake up to the fact that they are more than observers. They come to terms with the knowledge that "tradition is a living process and not merely passing on of inert objects."[13] They begin to understand themselves as agents of the tradition, stewards of the living, dynamic, and cumulative heritage entrusted to them. They are not involved in a handoff; they are an integral part of a vital process, the instrument of a throbbing reality that "exists from out of the present 'now' towards our future."[14]

Thus the formation process affirms and consolidates the leaders' professional identity. Leaders are called to mediate the practical wisdom and spiritual values of a "community of memory and tradition."[15] They assume responsibility for the stories, symbols, and metaphors of the Catholic Health Care ministry. And they identify themselves with a specific understanding of human life and destiny.

Over three years, our participants work out the implications of their theologically grounded, faith-based identity.

A Pluralistic Society: Who Will Lead?

To assert that anyone who leads a Catholic Health Care ministry needs a faith-based professional identity grounded in call gives rise to some serious questions that demand theological answers. The remainder of this chapter will address an important issue that requires analysis: religious pluralism and leadership within the context of the Catholic Health Care ministry. This issue brings up many questions: How can persons who are not Catholic, who belong to another faith or system of meaning, lay claim to Catholic identity? What is the nature of their relationship to the Church in general and the healing ministry of Jesus in particular? What does it mean to be called and who is called to the healing ministry?[16] In the end, might it be appropriate to give preference to Catholic candidates for senior leadership positions? Why? Why not?

Although non-Catholic leaders are widely accepted and well respected, there has been no compelling case from within the tradition itself to explicate their status theologically. It seems both unfair and unwise to leave this theological territory unexplored.

One might say that these questions are hypothetical. Many senior leaders in Catholic Health Care are indeed other-than-Catholic. This may be true; but often the situation has resulted because of supply and demand in leadership selection rather than intentional choice. Although non-Catholic leaders are widely accepted and well respected, there has been no compelling case from within the tradition itself to explicate their status theologically. It seems both unfair and unwise to leave this theological territory unexplored, since every leader in ministry, Catholic or not, needs and deserves validation from within the tradition he or she has pledged to serve.

The Second Vatican Council, a gathering of the world's Roman Catholic bishops (1962–1965), inaugurated a distinctive development in the Church's self-understanding. Several key Vatican II documents are directly relevant to our theological exploration.

Early in the Council's deliberations, the Belgian Cardinal Leo Jozef Suenens introduced the critical distinction between the Church *ad intra* and the Church *ad extra*. He insisted that the conciliar deliberations and documents focus on both the inner life of the Church (*ad intra*) and its engagement in the world (*ad extra*).[17] Suenens's distinction led to the publication of two important documents on the Church, the *Dogmatic Constitution on the Church* (*Lumen Gentium*), which for the most part focuses on the internal life of the Church, and the *Pastoral Constitution on the Church in the Modern World* (*Gaudium et Spes*), which reflects upon the Church's active presence in the modern world. Two other conciliar documents—the *Decree on Ecumenism* and the *Declaration on the Relationship of the Church to Non-Christian Religions*—are also relevant to our reflection concerning the theological implications of ministry leaders who are not Catholic.

Vatican II was pastoral and ecumenical. It presented an ecclesiology—a way of thinking about the Church—that emphasized self-renewal as well as dialogue and the Church's need to "read the signs of the times." The focus was on "motivating Christians to act together and singly in service to the whole world, through dialogue and cooperation with *all* persons of good will."[18] The Council very intentionally directed its message at *all* Christians and *all* persons of good will, not just Catholics.[19]

Vatican II marked the beginning of a new era in the relation of the Catholic Church to non-Catholic Christians and their ecclesial communities. In the *Decree on Ecumenism*, the Council recognizes that non-Catholic Christians participate in the life of the Church and that many of "the most significant elements or endowments which together go to build up and give life to the Church herself can exist outside the visible boundaries of the Catholic Church."[20] The decree calls for respect and affection in recognizing that all baptized persons are brought into a certain communion with the Catholic Church. The Catholic Church acknowledges that non-Catholic Christians share much of what in the past was viewed as strictly the *ad intra* possession of the Catholic Church, despite their not being in full ecclesiastical communion: "Baptism, therefore, constitutes a sacramental bond of unity linking all who have been reborn by means of it."[21]

Here we find a partial answer to the questions already posed regarding the relationship of those who are not Catholic to the healing ministry of Jesus Christ: all baptized persons participate in the life of the Church. The Council stresses that all Christians participate in "a life of grace." All Christians, Catholic or not, are called "to work together in the use of every possible means to relieve the afflictions of our times, such as famine and natural disasters, illiteracy and poverty."[22] Can there be any doubt that a well-motivated, non-Catholic, Christian leader and her Catholic colleagues in the healing ministry share a common identity grounded in Jesus Christ? *Lumen Gentium* clearly dispels any such doubt: "We can say that in some real way they are joined with us in the Holy Spirit, for to them also He gives His gifts and graces, and *is thereby operative among them.*"[23]

Excluding well-motivated, non-Catholic Christians from leadership in a Catholic Health Care ministry would be theologically baseless and misguided. Market realities in any case make inclusion of these leaders inescapable. All Christians hear the selfsame call in Jesus Christ. They may not inhabit the same ecclesiastical boundaries; yet, the source and center of their calling is identical to their Catholic brothers and sisters. The thought of excluding them from the Church's healing ministry conjures up the closing line of *Romeo and Juliet*: "All are punished!" And the suitability of including them underscores the need for excellent ministry leadership programs, where they can integrate and learn to articulate a specifically Catholic understanding of the Church's approach to the healing ministry against the background of their own baptismal call.

We must now peel back the next layer: How are we to understand the relationship of non-Christian leaders to the healing ministry of Jesus? Theologically speaking, how can those coming from another faith or system of meaning be "called"? In what way might their identity within a Catholic organization be viewed as "faith-based"? Here we can turn to the highly original *Declaration on the Relationship of the Church to Non-Christian Religions* as well as to the Church's traditional teaching on God's relationship to the world.

Vatican II hails the spiritual and moral goods found within non-Christian religions: "The Catholic Church rejects nothing which is true and holy in these religions. She looks with sincere respect upon those ways of conduct and of life, those rules and teachings which, though differing in many particulars from what she holds and sets forth, nevertheless often reflect a ray of that Truth which enlightens all men."[24] The Church here asserts that non-Christian religions possess elements of authentic truth. Moreover, the Church encourages Catholics "to prudently and lovingly through dialogue and collaboration" learn to appreciate and, where appropriate, draw upon the moral values and practical wisdom of non-Christian traditions.[25] Put somewhat differently, we should from time to time escape the bounds of our "homogeneous, closed spiritual landscapes."[26] This receptive attitude reveals more than an open spirit; it bespeaks theological conviction about God and God's relationship to humankind.

The Church's theological understanding of God's relationship to humankind, that is, its theological anthropology, emphasizes the idea of the human person created in the image and likeness of God. It further holds that each person is capable of knowing and loving the Creator.[27] All men and women are called into relationship with their Creator.[28] This is the source of the Church's feeling of deep solidarity with the human race and its history.[29] It is here in the Church's view of the human person that we shall find additional perspective on the questions under consideration.

We now return to the distinction between *ad intra* and *ad extra*. We noted that Cardinal Suenens had used this distinction to underscore the Church's need for a bifocal approach, that is, a need to look both within itself and beyond itself to its relations with the world. Cardinal Suenens had borrowed the distinction from a much earlier period (the fourth century), when it was first used to distinguish between the inner-directed (*ad intra*) and the outer-directed (*ad extra*) relationships of the Trinity, that is, Father, Son, and Holy Spirit.

Be assured! We will not wander off into the intricacies of Trinitarian theology at this point! Following a quick description, we will turn immediately to practical application in the present context. Generally speaking, the discussion of the Trinity *ad intra* focuses upon the relations between the divine persons—Father, Son, and Holy Spirit—*within* the Godhead, while the consideration of the Trinity *ad extra* focuses on the manner in which God enters into the human situation. In discussing the relationship of non-Christians to the healing ministry of Jesus Christ, we are concerned with the *ad extra* workings of God, that is, how we understand God's communication with us in time and history.

As we have seen, the Church teaches that God has reached out to humanity in Jesus Christ. In the Christian tradition Jesus is the Call incarnate, God among us. St. Paul uses the Greek term *kalon*, "the one who calls," in referring to Jesus. Christians are called by God in and through Jesus Christ, who "fully reveals humanity to itself and brings to light its very high calling."[30] In Jesus, God "'utters' himself outwards" (*ad extra*).[31]

That is all well and good, but what about the vast majority of men and women who are supposedly blind to His revelation and deaf to His call? How might non-Christians be called? And how could they assume a faith-based identity? The answer lies in understanding the *ad extra* relationship of God to humankind, that is, how the Church believes that God addresses each person in his or her own time and place. We shall see that God's *ad extra* self-communication "occurs in *two* basic ways which belong together," namely, through the Word of Jesus and also through the Love of the Holy Spirit.[32]

In his first encyclical, Pope Paul VI, who presided over the close of the Second Vatican Council, provides a simple yet eloquent way of describing the back and forth between the divine and human. He refers to it in terms of dialogue. And he is unequivocally inclusive in describing its scope: the dialogue "was made accessible to all; it was destined for all without distinction."[33] He further recognized that the dynamic interplay between God and human beings, "a many splendored conversation,"[34] takes place on different levels or planes, "consisting of a series of concentric circles around the central point in which God has placed us."[35]

God reaches out (*ad extra*) to those who dwell in the concentric circles of the human family. Paul VI describes the first of these circles as the whole of humanity, the second as those who embrace various forms of religion, and the third as the circle of Christianity. Following Paul VI, Pope John Paul II adopted the image of concentric circles and expressed appreciation for Paul VI's ability to heighten the awareness of the Church throughout the world, that is, within the first circle: "I keep thanking God that this great Predecessor of mine, who was also truly my father, knew how to display *ad extra*, externally, the true countenance of the Church."[36] In this context, John Paul II used the term *ad extra*, proposed by Cardinal Suenens at the Second Vatican Council, in simply referring to the Church's external relationship to the world. It was not intended as *ad extra* in the theological, Trinitarian sense, which focuses upon how "God freely steps outside himself" and into the human situation.[37] But John Paul II did not underestimate the importance of Paul VI's *ad extra* display of Christ and His Church to the world: "These words are listened to also by non-Christians. The life of Christ speaks, also, to many who are not capable of repeating with Peter: 'You are the Christ, the Son of the living God.' He, the Son of the living God, speaks to people also as Man: it is his life that speaks, his humanity, his fidelity to the truth, his all-embracing love."[38] People can and do find inspiration in the life and ministry of Jesus. As people of good will, they identify with Jesus' good intentions and may even decide to imitate his inspiring care and concern for others, even if they do not become Christians. They are attracted. Might an implicit note of call be detected here?

In any case, there is a deeper, universal source of calling for all non-Christians, even if they have never heard of Jesus. As John Paul II insisted, there "is the indwelling of God in each human being," which provides the radical link between us and our Creator.[39] Thus, he was deeply committed to exploring the more technical, theological, Trinitarian understanding of *ad extra*, the movement from within God to the world. ·

> It has been generally recognized that John Paul II's main theme is the indwelling of God in each human being and consequently in human society. . . . It is the spiritual reality of God's indwelling that pervades the twelve encyclicals he wrote. It is the basis of practically all he writes on the role of the Trinity and of Jesus Christ in the life of a human being. . . . He stresses that the acknowledgement of this divine presence in every human being is the way the church has to follow.[40]

Here, in the profoundly Trinitarian theology of John Paul II, we will find answers to our question regarding those leaders of Catholic ministries who are not Christian. Again, we need not enter into an extended discussion of Trinitarian theology. The point is straightforward. As we have said, God's *ad extra* self-communication occurs in two basic ways which belong together, namely, through the Word of Jesus and also through the Love of the Holy Spirit.[41] Although not everyone hears the explicit call in Christ, the entire human family can hear and respond to its gentle echo in the Holy Spirit, "the 'hidden God,' who as love and gift 'fills the universe.'"[42]

The action of the Holy Spirit grounds "God's presence in the intimacy of the human being, in mind, conscience, and heart."[43] In his encyclical *Lord and Giver of Life*, John Paul II spells it out:

> we need to go further back to even before the Christ if we want to embrace the whole of the action of the Holy Spirit throughout the world. For this action has been exercised in every place and at every time, indeed in every individual, also "outside the visible body of the church," as the Second Vatican Council reminds us, speaking precisely of "all people of good will in whose hearts grace works in an unseen way. For, since Christ died for all, and since the ultimate vocation of the human being is in fact one and divine, we ought to believe that the Holy Spirit in a manner known only to God offers every human being the possibility of being associated with the paschal mystery" [that is, the work of Jesus Christ].[44]

Pope Benedict XVI draws the inevitable conclusion in writing that all "human persons are the beings who can be Jesus Christ's brothers and sisters" and that "we must look upon them as persons who are called, together with us."[45] They may or may not find their way to the fullness of the call that "was made visible in Christ," but they do have a share in the ultimate human vocation that invites each of us to live a life based on goodness and love.[46] "The human being," says Benedict XVI, "is directly related to God. The human being is called."[47]

Non-Christians are thus called. Like Christians, they are invited to embrace the quest for truth, goodness, and love. In view of God's universal "presence in the intimacy of the human being, in mind, conscience, and heart," non-Christians are formally recognized as potential brothers and sisters of Christ. Like all human beings, they are in the most fundamental sense called to love and service through God's *ad extra* self-communication in the creative act. Thus, although they may not be formally bound to the Church through baptism, their capacity and in many cases sincere desire to join with the Church in its own *ad extra* activities (ministries) come "naturally." As Vatican II noted, "even if they have not arrived at an explicit knowledge of God,"[48] all people of good will are called to join with the Church "in her task to uncover, cherish, and ennoble all that is true, good, and beautiful in the human community."[49] On this most fundamental level of call, we can then find no formal theological reason to exclude those coming from another faith or system of meaning from senior leadership roles in Catholic Health Care ministries.

They are in full possession of the universal call addressed to each of us by the Creator. They bear the indelible imprint of God's image.[50] Their leadership capacity and commitment ought be understood as flowing from the all-embracing *ad extra* love of the Creator, "the grace-giving partner" who "has summoned forth humanity's beginning" and sustains its creative energies.[51]

Although we have exposed the theological bedrock that in principle supports a leadership role in Catholic Health Care for those coming from another faith or system of meaning, the picture is still incomplete. A principled theological argument for inclusion should not infer uncritical acceptance.

"For many are called, but few are chosen."[52] When Jesus uttered these words, he was not speaking about some arbitrary decision about who is in and who is out. And he really was not focused on the numbers—whether few or many. Rather, he was addressing the basic disposition of those who would authentically identify with his message and mission. As we have said, the capacity to join the

Church in its own *ad extra* activities (ministries) comes "naturally," that is, it is guaranteed by the deeper *ad extra* love of the creator for humanity. But innate capacity must be augmented by a clear line of personal and professional development that demonstrates compatibility with the organizational and moral demands of leadership within a Catholic Health Care ministry.

John C. Haughey sees this *call* through the lens of conversion. Haughey refers to the universal call addressed to us in creation as a "conversion to reality." Again, it comes naturally "into our consciousness through our senses and understandings."[53] On this level, people "are being true to their calls by seeking to know the truth in the myriad daily little and big ways *it* continually addresses them."[54] The *it*, of course, is the Spirit.

On another level, call becomes more specific and, for our purposes, very instructive. On the one hand, it provides a link between the generalized call embedded in each of human being by the Creator, and on the other hand it highlights the distinctive calling of those who lead Catholic Health Care ministries. This second way "to understand call is as a conversion to the ever-unfolding good, to the ways of being and doing that are seen as the right and valuable way of choosing to be."[55] According to Haughey, this level involves "hearing the call to live meaningfully, as this is construed through the meaning-making communities of which one is part."[56]

Assuming the universal ground of possibility offered in God's freely stepping outside himself (*ad extra*), anyone who responds specifically to the call to live meaningfully and authentically and embraces the Catholic Health Care ministry as a meaning-making community moves into an orbit of congeniality and commitment that requires a thankful, positive response. And, if as the gravitational pull becomes stronger, a person expressly commits to the healing ministry and consistently exhibits leadership gifts that promote the mission, vision, and moral values of the ministry, why would they be denied consideration for a senior leadership position? This would be more than hypocrisy; it would constitute an affront to the Catholic tradition, which sees the *ad extra* projection of God's image in each person and clearly affirms the view that includes non-Christians "in the fulfillment of the divine plan of salvation that God established in Christ and through the Church."[57] As the *ad extra* expression of God's love, they have a rightful place in the *ad extra* ministry of the Church because they freely allow this tradition to shape their horizon of meaning and willingly enter into a transformative culture that touches them deeply and informs their professional behavior. *In sum, then, given the proper disposition, requisite formation, professional gifts, and sustained commitment, those who come from another faith or system of meaning must be deemed worthy leaders and potential exemplars within the Catholic Health Care ministry. As leaders, they are in every way comparable to those who enjoy the mark of baptism.*[58]

Given the proper disposition, requisite formation, professional gifts, and sustained commitment, those who come from another faith or system of meaning must be deemed worthy leaders and potential exemplars within the Catholic Health Care ministry.

Conclusion

Within the context of ministry formation, theology must always be running in the background. Each element in the program and every step in the process require attention to the underlying theological rationale that gives direction and substance to the overall project. An invitational design, adult orientation, theological expertise, and a dialogical method may appear as discrete elements in a programmatic game plan. Further, a theological reflection on who may or may not qualify to lead a Catholic Health Care ministry might seem like an interesting add-on. Yet, this chapter represents a consistent line of insight and inspiration that would seem to suggest otherwise.

As noted earlier, the Ministry Leadership Formation Program is more than an academic enterprise; it serves as a living link between the teachings of the Catholic Christian tradition and a world of culture in continuous development. As such, the Center is part of the theological enterprise itself. Consequently, each element of the program is in service to a deeper, theological *raison d'etre*. The invitational design, for example, clears resistance to addressing theological concerns and allows the emergence of an unembarrassed attachment to core theological concerns of the Catholic tradition. Consequently, most participants are generally comfortable engaging in theological

> Within the context of ministry formation, theology must always be running in the background. Each element in the program and every step in the process require attention to the underlying theological rationale that gives direction and substance to the overall project.

reflection concerning the tradition; and through this reflection and their subsequent action, tradition is renewed and spilled into the world of health care.

In a similar vein, our adult orientation moves into the real world, where theological niceties do not cut it. The theological perspective on suffering, for instance, must address the lived experience of the mature executive who is looking for a meaningful link between raw suffering and their own calling. Our adult orientation encourages us to stand back while participants "inhabit their own suffering." We are not there to teach in the strict sense, but we are there to witness and theologize as we facilitate—or perhaps mediate—the richness of the tradition and what it has to offer in the practical order of participant experience. In other words, we function as guides who can offer theological perspective that is respectful and oriented toward practice. The theology of hope, for example, has proved very relevant to the day-to-day experience of many participants as they confront suffering in themselves, their colleagues, and the people they serve. In the reservoir of the tradition's view of hope, they report having found a new courage and a more or less effective antidote to the anxiety they experience on a daily basis. A rather complex theological category has been appropriated at a very basic, practical level. Truly, the adult learner's dream!

And, as we have explained, our dialogical method of the Triangle lies at the heart of the formation enterprise. The Triangle is the engine of theological reflection that allows the Center to fulfill its mission to conserve, explicate, and transmit Catholicism's rich heritage to those entrusted with the Church's health care ministries.

The foregoing discussion highlights the essentially theological nature of ministry leadership formation. Our work is not about leadership per se, nor is it an exercise in personal and professional development. Our aim is nothing less than *personal and organizational transformation* within and through a community of memory and meaning. Within the extended context of the formation experience, individuals are invited to reformulate—or in many cases simply reinforce—their worldview by aligning themselves and their organizations with the theological impulse that guides the health care ministry, namely, the conviction that "the act of personal love for another human being is . . . the all-embracing basic act of humankind which gives meaning, direction, and measure to everything else."[59]

We have moved through some fairly rugged theoretical, theological terrain. One can only hope that it has not been a path too complicated or too abstract. Even a winding path, though, often leads to a clearing in the woods. Here, within the open space of our concluding paragraphs, we feel compelled to offer some personal testimony.

After eight years of working with more than seven hundred executives, we can unequivocally state that the Catholic Health Care ministry is in good hands. These executives represent the complex, rich culture of the United States. They are a rainbow of race, religion, philosophical perspective, personal preference, and leadership style. Yet, they share a common commitment to the Catholic Health Care ministry. The depth of their concern and their willingness to confront the economic and moral challenges associated with delivering distinctively Catholic services in a threatening environment exceeds any reasonable expectation. Yes, the wonderful communities of women and men religious who founded these exceptional health care institutions lived a special form of communal life; but the women and men who now take up the torch are no less unified and conformed to the same fundamental ideal. We have found in them an identifiable, indeed palpable, streak of determination to assume responsibility for the ministries entrusted to them. They believe! They enthusiastically enter the formation process, seeking a deeper understanding and practical direction for the day-to-day management of their institutions. This chapter sketches the inclusive Catholic theology that supports and gratefully embraces this "many splendored"[60] community of committed leaders within an "ecclesiology of friendship."[61] The first decade of the twenty-first century attests to the ministry's resilience. We are showing that it is possible to retain the tradition "not as the preservation of ashes, but as the feeding of a fire."[62]

Notes

1. Pope Paul VI, *On the Development of Peoples* (1967), section 67. All translations of the papal encyclicals in this chapter are from the Papal Encyclicals Online website.

2. Pope Benedict XVI, *God is Love* (2005), section 31c.

3. Pope Paul VI, *Paths of the Church* (1964), section 87.

4. Pope John Paul II, *On the Relationship between Faith and Reason* (Boston: Pauline Books, 1998), 10.

5. Hans Kung, *Christianity and World Religions* (New York: Orbis Books, 1993), xix.

6. Laurence J. O'Connell and John Shea, "Ministry Leadership Formation: Engaging with Leaders," *Health Progress*, September-October 2009, 34–39.

7. Our approach resonates with the changing style in general management

culture, where there is now discussion of "organizational conversation." See Boris Groysberg and Michael Slind, "Leadership Is a Conversation," *Harvard Business Review*, June 2012, 76–84.

8. The work of John Henry Newman represents the classic description of the Triangle's underlying principles. See John Henry Newman, *Essay on the Development of Christian Doctrine*, 6th ed. (South Bend: University of Notre Dame Press, 1988).

9. James D. Whitehead and Evelyn Eaton Whitehead, *Method in Ministry: Theological Reflection and Christian Ministry* (New York: Seabury Press, 1980); Whitehead and Whitehead, *Method in Ministry: Theological Reflection and Christian Ministry*, rev. ed. (Lanham, Md.: Sheed and Ward, 1995). For background on developments in the field of practical theology, see Don S. Browning, *A Fundamental Practical Theology* (Minneapolis: Augsburg Fortress, 1991); and Richard R. Osmer, *Practical Theology* (Grand Rapids, Mich.: William B. Eerdmans, 2008).

10. Pope John Paul II, *On the Relationship between Faith and Reason*, section 107.

11. Jan Walgrave, *Unfolding Revelation: The Nature of Doctrinal Development* (Philadelphia: Westminster, 1972), 41.

12. William Cox, "Nurturing the Ministry's Soul," *Health Progress*, September-October 2004, 38–43.

13. Walgrave, *Unfolding Revelation*, 40.

14. Karl Rahner, *Foundations of Christian Faith*, ed. William Dych (New York: Herder and Herder, 1972), 431. See also Pope Paul VI, *Paths of the Church*, 25: "The Church needs to reflect on herself. She needs to feel the throb of her own life."

15. Browning, *A Fundamental Practical Theology*, 2.

16. See Laurence J. O'Connell, "Vocation," in *The Dictionary of Catholic Spirituality*, ed. Michael Downey (Collegeville, Minn.: Liturgical Press, 1993), 1009–1010; Laurence J. O'Connell, "Towards a Theology of Vocation," *Chicago Studies* 18 (1979): 147–159.

17. Giuseppe Albergio, *A Brief History of Vatican II* (New York: Orbis Books, 2005), 29–30, 122.

18. Richard McBrien, *The Church: The Evolution of Catholicism* (New York: HarperCollins, 2009), 196.

19. Walter M. Abbott, ed., *The Documents of Vatican II* (New York: America Press, 1966), 2–7.

20. Ibid., 345.

21. Ibid., 364.

22. Ibid., 355.

23. Ibid., 34 (emphasis my own).

24. Ibid., 662.

25. Ibid.

26. Karl Rahner, *Theological Investigations* (London: Darton, Longman & Todd, 1969), 6:34. John Haughey amplifies this point in his stimulating discussion of the virtue of hospitality in the Church's ministries: "The Church has to learn how to host the work of God taking place not only within but also outside the borders of its own self-understanding and institutions." John Haughey, *Where Is God Going* (Washington, D.C.: Georgetown University Press, 2009), 35.

27. Abbott, *Documents of Vatican II*, 210.

28. Ibid., 30.

29. Ibid., 400.

30. Ibid., 220.

31. Karl Rahner, *The Trinity* (London: Burns & Oates, 1970), 89.

32. Ibid., 88.

33. Paul VI, *Paths of the Church*, section 76.

34. Ibid., section 70.

35. Ibid., section 96.

36. John Paul II, *Redemptor Hominis*, section 4.

37. Rahner, *The Trinity*, 86.

38. John Paul II, *Redemptor Hominis*, section 4.

39. Joseph G. Donders, ed., *John Paul II: The Encyclicals in Everyday Language* (New York: Orbis Books, 2005), ix–x.

40. Ibid.

41. Rahner, *The Trinity*, 88.

42. Donders, *John Paul II: The Encyclicals*, 102.

43. Ibid.

44. Ibid.

45. Joseph Ratziger, *"In the Beginning . . .": A Catholic Understanding of the Story of Creation and the Fall* (Grand Rapids, Mich.: William B. Eerdmans, 1995), 48–49.

46. Donders, *John Paul II: The Encyclicals*, 54.

47. Ratzinger, *"In the Beginning,"* 45.

48. Abbott, *Documents of Vatican II*, 35.

49. Ibid., 289.

50. See the Apostolic Letter *Porta Fidei*, issued by Pope Benedict XVI on October 11, 2011, section 10.

51. Rahner, *Theological Investigations*, 6:11, 20.

52. Matthew 22:14.

53. John C. Haughey, ed., *Revisiting the Idea of Vocation: Theological Explorations* (Washington, D.C.: Catholic University of America Press, 2004), 3.

54. Ibid., 4.

55. Ibid.

56. Ibid., 1.

57. Richard McBrien, *The Church*, 22.

58. In fact, the Second Vatican Council warns against those who would assume that baptized Christians might take precedence, since some Christians "remain indeed in the bosom of the Church, but, as it were, only in 'bodily' manner and not 'in his or her heart.'" *Lumen Gentium*, 14. *Baptism cannot be the determining factor in who may or may not lead a Catholic Health Care ministry.* A simple external sign cannot trump authentic internal disposition. A ministry leader may accept his or her call "silently but nevertheless genuinely; or to use St. Augustine's formula regarding the Church: some think they are 'inside' when in terms of their own truth they are really 'outside,' and some consider themselves or are considered to be 'outside' when in reality they are 'inside.'" Rahner, *Theological Investigations*, 6:41.

59. Rahner, *Theological Investigations*, 6:241.

60. Paul VI, *Paths of the Church*, section 70.

61. John D. Dabosky, "Towards a Fundamental Theological Re-Interpretation of Vatican II," *Heythrop Journal* 49, no. 5 (September 2008): 742–763.

62. Avery Dulles, *Models of the Church* (New York: Doubleday, 1974), 60.

CHAPTER 4

The Relationship between Leadership Development and Leadership Formation

Andre L. Delbecq

Most individuals occupying leadership positions in contemporary organizations understand the concept of leadership development. Programs may differ by level or function, for example, they may be supervisory, managerial, executive, staff, marketing, or accounting. However, in all cases most would describe leadership development as an educational experience emphasizing managerial and organizational skills that contribute to the effective exercise of leadership. Leadership development differs from "pre-entry" education such as an MBA program in its pedagogy (participatory adult learning by in-role leaders), contextualization (tailoring to a particular organization and its mission), and utilization of immediate organizational experience as an essential part of the learning design.

Organizationally sponsored leadership formation is less well understood. Individual spiritual formation is more familiar. Traditionally, spiritual formation referenced a program of spiritual development and guidance for those called to a deep religious life (pastor, priest, clergyperson, rabbi, nun, and so on). However, at the beginning of this new century, spirituality has emerged as a mega-trend. Spiritual formation for "lay" persons fully involved in modern life within secular institutions is also a robust development. Most spiritual formation programs are housed within a religious tradition (Buddhism, Christianity, Judaism, Hinduism, Muslim, and so on) or offered through religiously plural spirituality centers.

Organizationally sponsored leadership formation is a form of spiritual formation wherein the focus is on the vocational calling of an organizational leader within the context of an organizational mission, for example, health care, higher education, or social services. Normally leaders move through the program as a "cohort." As is the case with leadership development, the program is richly contextualized to an organizational mission and setting. Likewise, the pedagogy is adult learning that uses shared reflection by participants and immediate organizational applications as important elements of the pedagogy. Although individual spiritual development and disciplines are included, reference is always returned to how a mature spirituality is enacted within the context of organizational leadership.

> Organizationally sponsored leadership formation is a form of spiritual formation wherein the focus is on the vocational calling of an organizational leader within the context of an organizational mission.

The purpose of this chapter is modest. It seeks to provide greater clarity regarding how leadership development and leadership formation differ, but also how they complement each other. It illustrates the relationship through the lens of four content areas characteristic of most leadership development programs. Through these parallel descriptions, the reader will come to greater clarity regarding the domain and contribution of leadership formation.

The Illustrative Topics

In this brief chapter we focus only through the important but limited lens of "content." (The reader should refer to other chapters for an exposition of pedagogy and learning designs.) We obviously cannot overview all topics characteristic of quality programs. Here we juxtapose leadership development with leadership formation using just four exemplary content areas: teamwork, decision-making, organization design and structure, and organizational culture.

Teamwork

A leader's relationship with individual associates is a major emphasis when dealing with the technical core of organizations. While individual relationships remain central regardless of organizational level, teams become a more dominant focal point for senior leaders. At upper organizational levels, leaders spend an increasing amount of their time dealing with strategic issues that transcend individual efforts. For senior leaders, problem and solution complexity requires the pooling of judgments within teams. Coordination across both internal and external boundaries requires teamwork to create linkages for effective implementation. Leadership must also facilitate teamwork surrounding visioning, problem-solving processes, and implementation efforts associated with innovation.

> While individual relationships remain central regardless of organizational level, teams become a more dominant focal point for senior leaders.

Typical topics addressed in a leadership development program regarding teamwork might include:

- the impact of size on effective teamwork;

- norms and processes for maintaining a collaborative culture within a team;

- membership challenges including recruiting, composition, and managing participant transitions;

- complementary leadership roles, that is, task leader, social emotional leader, process facilitator, and so on;

120

- stages of team functioning such as forming, establishing norms, and engaging action;

- the centrality of carefully mandated and focused team goals;

- managing team meeting agendas;

- conflict resolution and decision processes appropriate for different team tasks;

- attention to outcomes, evaluation, and double-loop learning; and

- exemplification of different forms of teamwork, that is, design, innovation, quality control, and so on.

Most readers of this chapter will have participated in some form of team-oriented leadership development, so these topics will resonate with their personal experience.

How would leadership formation enrich the discussion of teamwork? The following themes associated with leadership formation provide examples of how this overlay has the potential to deepen effective leadership for teamwork. Here we have space to only reference a Christian perspective through the lens of five topics. Many of the themes that follow find echoes across spiritual traditions: the dignity of individuals; the nature of calling and charism; the importance of community; the virtues of patience, forgiveness, courage, hopefulness, and so on in support of community; overarching mission. In the Christian tradition the dignity of each person is a sine qua non of leadership formation. The tradition is clear: we must recognize the presence of the divine in each person and treat him or her with respect and love. This is not the "luv" of hallmark cards but rather a deep abiding respect that welcomes each person, including any flaws that are part of human nature. Thus, the theology of the individual person, so central within leadership formation, will influence the tone of a leader's relation with other team players. Being accepted not simply for contribution, role, or skill but rather as a whole person frees a team participant from trying to prove or compete. This increases the probability that the team can focus on "contribution to mission" without the distraction of a need for posturing by individual team members.

Further, leadership formation in the Christian tradition posits the belief that each individual is called by name, in his or her individuality with his or her unique differences, to contribute to noble efforts on behalf of others. A formation program explores how each person possesses differentiated charisms, gifts of the Holy Spirit given for the benefit of the community. A spiritually mature leader is alert to the manifestation of these gifts among the members of a team, calls them forth, and expresses gratitude for them. Thus, the leader is not threatened by or envious of the gifts of others. Having your individuality honored and your gifts recognized by a leader is a powerful motivator for team members that positively changes the dynamics of decision-making as we will see in the discussion of decision-making.

> Being accepted not simply for contribution, role, or skill but rather as a whole person frees participants from trying to prove or compete. This increases the probability that the team can focus on "contribution to mission" without the distraction of a need for posturing by individual team members.

The deep internalization of the universal concept of calling, deeper than job (a series of tasks) or career (a series of moves through roles), is an essential component in leadership formation. A leader too is called by name, and leadership is understood as a particular charism. Leadership is conceived as servant leadership, not the aggrandizement of power, prestige, or competitive advantage. Further, since the charism of leadership is understood as given on behalf of others, the leader must always orient team efforts toward the larger others whom the organization serves. Thus, the energies of a team are directed away from individual member or group advantage toward a greater common good. This is a vital protection against a team becoming a self-serving clique.

Community is another central topic in leadership formation. In the Christian tradition we are called to community by the very nature of the Triune Mystery of the Trinity. As noted earlier, a mature spiritual understanding of community accepts the humanity of each participant including human weakness. It understands human nature as fallen and does not feast on flaws or unduly lament human imperfection. It understands why gossip and detraction are considered primary offenses against community in the monastic traditions. But it also understands human nature as saved, and so the role of a spiritually mature leader is to aid all members of a team to strive toward greater light and greater degrees of human perfection even while being aware that imperfect persons accomplish important outcomes through grace. Patience, forbearance, hopefulness, and a sense of humor mark the graduate of a leadership formation program as opposed to cynicism, discouragement, and burnout. Formed leaders realize that teamwork within organizations demands special sensitivities toward each individual, but also is concerned with the team becoming a supportive community.

It takes a spiritually mature leader to remain focused on a contributory goal, a goal that is focused on the well-being of those who are served, which includes paying attention to individuals who might otherwise be marginalized.

The requirements for pooled problem solving in complex contemporary settings often require heterogeneous teams where membership is differentiated by function, career stage, background, and so on. Empirically such groups are difficult to bring into cohesion. They require patience, a willingness to remain in long periods of uncertainty, the need to avoid distractions created by individual differences, and so on. The spiritually formed leader understands that virtuous leadership behavior is required in such difficult circumstances.

123

Studies of teamwork emphasize a focused goal as a distinguishing condition for effective teamwork. But not all goals are equal. Organizational members typically identify with the overarching organizational mission. But how this mission is refracted in a design group, an audit team, a compensation committee, a quality control group, and so on is often less clear. It is easy for an overall noble purpose to be corrupted by self-serving advantage, sub-optimization, undue competitiveness, and so on. The leader needs to be able to continually assist a group to test its unfolding processes against ultimate concerns. Yet spiritually immature leaders often regress to comparative or competitive benchmarks. It takes a spiritually mature leader to remain focused on a contributory goal, a goal that is focused on the well-being of those who are served, which includes paying attention to individuals who might otherwise be marginalized. A hallmark of leadership formation is attention to noble organizational purpose, always sifting and winnowing group behavior and outcomes consistent with mission.

The spiritually immature team leader is often insecure and fearful, seeks protection of the false self through controlling and hyper-competitive behavior, and preys on individual member imperfections. Spiritual formation makes a difference.

Still, leadership formation is not simply knowledge of desirable behavior. Formation must help form habits of the heart brought to maturity through spiritual practice. An un-centered leader, primarily concerned with personal preference, impatient with others, and unforgiving of individual weaknesses, an egoistic leader who has not engaged in spiritual practice that would thereby mitigate the mischief of the false self, is unlikely to successfully guide a team in difficult times. Therefore, leadership formation not only provides a refracted worldview. It also provides a path. It serves as a laboratory for the personal appropriation of spiritual practices that enable continued growth toward spiritual maturity. Spiritual disciplines of prayer, reflection, and meditation engender spiritual growth that is more capable of deep listening, holding antinomies, negotiating conflict resolution, and so on. Thus, it is not only what the leader understands about how one should normatively proceed when guiding complex team endeavors that underlies leadership formation. Spiritual leadership also requires an inner conversion and openness to transcendence, which is achieved only through spiritual practices. So in the end the leader's inner spiritual growth is also a litmus test of a quality leadership formation program. Good programs are evaluated by self-perceived behavior changes but also attested to by perceptions of organizational associates.

Pause and contrast this portrayal of a spiritually formed team leader to simply a skilled but spiritually immature team leader. The spiritually immature team leader is often insecure and fearful, seeks the protection of the false self through controlling and hyper-competitive behavior, and preys on individual member imperfections. Spiritual formation makes a difference.

Decision-Making

A leader is measured by the quality of decisions arrived at. At lower levels leaders serve as experts and so individual decision-making is prominent. However, as discussed earlier, increasingly at all levels and particularly at senior levels, the role of the leader is to manage a decision-making process that is inclusive of others requiring the pooling of judgments in order to arrive at strategic solutions. Here we will focus on "strategic decisions," where both the nature of the problem and the elements of the solution need to be discovered over time. This genre of decision is most important to senior leaders and most prone to decision failure.

Typical topics in a leadership development program dealing with decision-making might include:

- categories of decisions: routine decisions, where means and ends are codified; creative decisions, where ends are known but means must be discovered; conflict resolution decisions, where means are proposed but ends are debated; strategic decisions, where both the nature of the problem and the solution outcomes must be discovered;

- individual and group cognitive and affective processes influencing decision-making;

- techniques for enhancing creativity, such as brainstorming, nominal groups, delphi pooling, and so on;

- techniques for solution search, both internal and external to the organizational, including contemporary technology;

- techniques for conflict resolution;

- utilization of outside experts, such as advisors, consultants, and experts;

- protocols for moving through an innovation sequence, such as visioning, problem exploration, solution search, experimentation, and implementation;

- normative decision processes that are part of an organization's culture; and

- typical sources of distortion and error.

Again it is likely that readers will have participated in some form of leadership development associated with effective decision-making.

To begin, it is important to note that more than half the time studies show that strategic decision-making in the very best contemporary organizations fails. Failure is associated with the tendency to regress to "expert" patterns of decision-making, that is, assuming from past experience and prior organizational practices. This leads to precipitous closure on a solution comfortable for the leader and the participants. Negative outcomes are also associated with failure to listen carefully to other stakeholder voices (those who will feel the impact of the decision, those who disagree with the decision, and those who will exercise authority in connection with the decision). Closing out these voices leads to premature closure with only limited options having been considered. The leader then engages in uncritical promotion of this early solution focused on personal preferences and those of select informants. In other instances, the search for lessons in the behavior of other organizations is truncated and experimental approaches and action learning are not engaged. All of these distortions are seen in the behavior of well-trained and skilled individuals. Obviously strategic decisions call for particularly elevated psychological and spiritual maturity.

> Discernment is a spiritual discipline that seeks freedom from subtle pressures that distort strategic decision-making for both individuals and organizational stakeholders.

What can leadership formation contribute to the avoidance of these pitfalls? We will discuss just three topics central to formation programs that bear on decision-making: the achievement of "indifference," the "beginner's mind" through meditative and contemplative practices; the criticality of patience and deep listening; and the classic discipline of discernment. Discernment is a spiritual discipline that seeks freedom from subtle pressures that distort strategic decision-making for both individuals and organizational stakeholders.

On any occasion when faced with a difficult problem, the human mind is subject to bias. The source of bias might be fear, a need for power, a tendency to compete, and the like. In our normal state of consciousness we are barely aware of these forces acting within our consciousness. Expert decision-making provides checklists and protocols in its codification of best practice to help a professional avoid such entrapments. But when we deal with strategic decision-making where ends and means must be discovered, often under conditions of organizational threat or performance downturns, these subconscious ghosts are particularly dangerous.

The normative state needed to deal with the unaware mind is clearly stated in the great traditions. For example, in the Christian tradition Ignatius of Loyola admonishes a need for "indifference," his term for being preference-free in seeking to discover the will of God and the well-being of those one serves. In the Buddhist tradition one speaks of the need for "emptiness" or the "beginner's mind." Of course, neither tradition believes that we can enter decision-making "without thoughts" or "without emotions." Rather, the great traditions understand that there is a need for spiritual disciplines that allow us to become aware of our deep inner thoughts and feelings, disciplines that allow the true self to be alert to potential distortion and find freedom to be open to truth. Spiritual disciplines of prayer, meditation, contemplation, and continual reexamination of consciousness and events gradually free individuals from the domination of mental distortions

A leader and a group that engage in discernment often experience unexpected insight and enlivened motivation that transcend prior knowing, leading to new courage and hopefulness.

that the undisciplined mind is hardly aware of. However, it is not just freedom from distortion but the inspiration of the Holy Spirit that is sought through discernment and its accompanying spiritual disciplines. Once the mind is stilled and intentions purified, another wisdom can be accessed, an enlightened way of knowing, understanding, and being present to the challenges. A leader and a group that engage in discernment often experience unexpected insight and enlivened motivation that transcend prior knowing, leading to new courage and hopefulness.

Strategic decision-making requires great patience and active learning throughout a long discovery process. It is fine to prescribe in decision theory that one should remain in the problem nexus without discomfort, but the false self is impatient and wants to resolve discomfort by premature actions. It is fine to prescribe deep listening to all stakeholder voices, but the false self prefers to listen to itself or some subset of favorite individuals. Thus, we see leaders tending to dominate, persuade, and force rather than creatively and patiently resolve conflicts.

As one moves through the complex sequences of strategic decision-making, we can trace the value of spiritual maturity at each step. When visioning, such maturity is open to creative re-conceptualization of ends and finds freedom to be concerned with noble purpose. When engaging in problem exploration with those who will feel the impact, such maturity is capable of deep listening and remaining centered on real, unresolved needs rather than provider or organizational convenience and preference. When exploring potential solution elements, such maturity is naturally open to incorporating the thinking of others, whether counsel comes from inside or outside the organization. Such maturity is comfortable with experimentation and the pilot testing of alternatives rather than the premature selection of a single course of action that tries to force its implementation on the organization. Such maturity welcomes double-loop learning and does not scapegoat innovation team members when things do not unfold as planned. Such maturity brings new resources to groups in difficulty and is able to be flexible when encountering setbacks and difficulties. In short, in every phase of strategic decision-making the spiritually mature leader has a greater openness to truth, a greater capacity for deep listening, greater patience, and a more generous willingness to incorporate the gifts of others. Leadership formation provides learning and spiritual disciplines that decrease the pitfalls so often reported in studies of strategic decision failure.

Thus, the discernment tradition overlays spiritual insight and supportive spiritual practices on sophisticated decision-making sequences. Further, leadership formation not only seeks to have a leader understand discernment but provides case situations and project contexts wherein discernment is experienced and practiced in the rough and tumble of complex organizational strategy.

Organization Design and Structure

Monocratic hierarchy with centralized command and control authority had been the dominant organization logic since the time of the pharaohs. Until very recently, whether in the military, the government, or the private sector, hierarchy with control centered in authority of office was the organizational form, which was modified in only limited ways by division of labor and specialization.

This is not the place to trace the revolution in organization design that has occurred and is becoming normative at the turn of the century. But increasing access to information, the required speed of decision-making, increased sub-specialization, and global competition have altered contemporary organization designs. When all of the evidence is taken together, leadership development programs make clear that a new model of contemporary organization is emerging. This new model is described as:

- flatter, with fewer levels of hierarchy;

- focused on quasi-autonomous, smaller, strategic business units that are empowered to respond quickly to the needs of differentiated market segments; accountable for their own efficiency and effectiveness; responsible for maintaining a capacity for rapid change and innovation inclusive of both new designs and continuous improvement innovation co-developed with client groups; expected to rapidly assimilate compatible changes brought from outside; allowed to gain share in resources they generate;

- where expert power increasingly plays an ever-larger role and where strategic decisions require the pooling of judgments;

- where teams are increasingly the dominant leadership forum;

- where the role of the leader is increasingly that of mentor, facilitator, and process guide rather than solo authority figure;

- where strategic business units are aggregated within large systems in order to achieve economies of scale through centralized service systems (e.g., information technology, centralized purchasing, and centralized capitalization); support from cadres of experts available in service to strategic business units; market and branding prominence; access to large capital resources; strategic environmental surveillance stimulating new endeavors; and strategic partnering.

Again readers will have participated in leadership development programs devoted to forms of organizational evolution occurring within their own environments. Macro-organizational change is a complex and rapidly evolving topic whereby the modern organization seeks to simultaneously gain the advantages of scale while maintaining the flexibility and spontaneity of smaller strategic business units unencumbered with undue bureaucratic overlays. Thereby, modern organization theory seeks to be bi-focal: giving attention to efficiencies and best practices (a degree of standardization) while giving freedom to units to manage continuous rapid change. Such a complex set of balances is no place for the psychologically and spiritually immature.

We will again suggest contributions from leadership formation here referencing only two topics: subsidiarity and community. The modern organizational setting with its great differentiation of structure and sub-unit foci requires significant conceptual flexibility. It is easy to sit in any single organizational location and from that sub-optimal seat be hypercritical of other organizational efforts. An individual in a clinical service (no matter how empowered the unit may be) will find decisions in his unit rubbing against pressures from a different unit's perspective. For example, the clinical unit will receive requests to accommodate large technical systems (Why can't we just use our own informal data? Purchase our own preferred supplies?), requests to meet stewardship goals (Why don't they cut costs elsewhere?), requests to engage new partners and clients in service to new market segments (Why can't we just concentrate on our own preferred clients?), and so on.

Subsidiarity sounds good in the abstract. The principle states that decisions should be made at the lowest possible level by people close to the problem (grounded in the lived experience of clients being served) and close to the solution elements (individuals with local knowledge, in-depth experience, and specialized training). Undue centralization and standardization, once seen as benchmarks of efficiency and effectiveness, now often create unnecessary "bureaucracy" (inflexibility, inefficiency, and added cost). Every contemporary leader spends considerable time buffering his subsidiary unit from undue pressures, whether these pressures arise from above or horizontally from centralized service units seeking economies of scale. At the same time, if an organizational unit wants the benefits of "largeness" (economies of scale and access to deep resources), it will have to integrate overall organizational efficiencies with empowered, decentralized units. The contemporary strategic unit's leader must manage this complex interface. As much as possible, a leader needs to protect a subsidiary unit from undue interference so it can rapidly and flexible serve its client base. At the same time, his or her unit will not be able to access resources if it is not integrated into the larger organizational whole, and it must be in service to the larger organizational purposes.

> A spiritually formed organizational leader must always be an advocate for the subsidiary rights of their unit participants, not simply an agent of seemingly innocuous changes that slowly but surely destroy the dignity and reduce the proper flexibility of those in a strategic business unit.

This places our earlier discussion of the skills required for mature "pooling of judgments" in a realistic context. In the modern organization, there are multiple stakeholders, differentiated preferences, varied problem logics (efficiency versus innovation), strong power bases, and strong egos. All the requirements of spiritual maturity, respect for each individual, appreciation for different gifts, and especially the continued need for discernment come into play.

Here the principle of subsidiarity discussed in leadership formation adds value. The normative preference to decentralize, empower, and trust associates in their legitimate sphere of decision-making is a critical anchor in formation programs. Organizational history is replete with examples of large organizations becoming calcified with undue bureaucracy and becoming over-controlled by individuals seeking to expand their power bases without this anchoring norm. Spontaneity, self-control, freedom to co-create, and motivation diminish under these circumstances. William White's "organization man" emerges, an associate simply putting in time in a dehumanized job where he or she feels other-directed and other-controlled. This is avoidable, of course. There are ways to achieve job enrichment, to increase individual creativity and self-control, and to enlist each associate's talents as a knowledge worker, whether on the front line (e.g., facilities maintenance) or at a senior level. But this requires constant vigilance by a graduate of a leadership formation program who is always alert to where subsidiarity is being unnecessarily violated and work is becoming less in keeping with human dignity. A spiritually formed organizational leader must always be an advocate for the subsidiary rights of their unit participants, not simply an agent of seemingly innocuous changes that slowly but surely destroy the dignity and reduce the proper flexibility of those in a strategic business unit.

We return to community as another important element for maintaining this difficult balance. Unless all the participants in a business unit feel they are an important part of the unit's noble purpose, and feel free to indicate discomfort and feel intuitively ill at ease with encroachments by other parts of the organization, their leader can easily slip into simply "working with the agents of change" (horizontally and vertically separate from the home unit). Soon such an immature leader fails to give voice to and be an advocate for the home unit. Indeed, a spiritually immature leader may concentrate on courting the favor of outside players, hoping by doing so to advance in career. Such a leader spends more and more time outside the home unit, losing touch with the just concerns and intuitions of those who are the leader's first responsibility.

We have artificially stressed one side of the argument for purposes of illustration. Of course there is the alternative distortion: failure to pay attention to the organizational common good because of an over-preoccupation with subunit convenience that leads to resistance to necessary change. Here other topics in leadership formation, including attention to the common good, concern with social justice, and a preferential option for the poor and marginalized, play an important role. There are no simple answers to balancing these concerns on the complex stage of the contemporary macro-organization. Thus, our continuing refrain regarding the needs for pooled judgments through careful and patient discernment. Only through such discernment can the leader arrive at decisions that honor the noble overall organizational purpose and at the same time provide dignity and appropriate subsidiary control within the organization.

In summary, subsidiarity as an organizational principle, while maintaining an open and participatory community (both central topics within leadership formation), provides important countervailing safeguards against either undue attention to macro-organizational logics at the expense of strategic unit needs or undue sub-optimal behavior with units. And yes, without prayer, meditation, and reflection, finding this Wisdom of Solomon is unlikely to occur.

Organizational Culture

We will close this chapter by discussing the topic of organizational culture. Organizational culture is usually defined as the deep but often subtle and implicit understandings about organizational purpose and acceptable behavior that shapes expectations among organizational members: "This is how we think about things here, go about doing things here, and also what we avoid doing if you want to accepted and rewarded here." Just saying "The IBM Way," "The Navy Way," or "The American Way" evokes a sense of differentiated culture.

Culture evolves over time as a result of many different factors. The typical leadership development program will address topics such as clarity of mission and values, normative codes of conduct, symbolic ways of right speaking, patterns that guide interpersonal and group relationships, systems of rewards and punishments, organizational rituals and rites of passage, founder stories and myths, memorable stories of success and failure, and symbols, art, and icons. Cultures are richly attended to by founders and in early years of organizational emergence. As the organization matures, culture becomes more implicit. Sometimes memories fade regarding why something is done in a certain way, but clear patterns that lead to an understanding that this is how things are done persist.

> Probably no topic receives more attention than mission and values in leadership formation programs.

Again most of us have participated in leadership development programs where culture is explored, leadership behavior that reinforces culture is explicated, and deep-culture organizations (Navy Seals, 3M, GE) are described.

What does leadership formation contribute to this final topic to be explored? Here we will reference the following topics included in formation programs: attention of mission and values, founder's stories, a sacramental and liturgical imagination, and challenges of religious pluralism. Probably no topic receives more attention than mission and values in leadership formation programs. The discussion is deeply rooted in a spiritual tradition (e.g., the healing ministry of Jesus in health care and forming men and women of conscience, competence, and compassion in Jesuit Higher Education). Formation understands how meaning in terms of ontological purpose is central to motivation. So the noble purpose of an organization expressed in spiritually rich language is explored and returned to over and over.

Founders' stories play a major role in leadership formation programs. The charisms of founders and their exceptional dedication to service as a form of "ministry," the hardships and struggles of their journey, and the importance of a supportive community as a critical element in sustaining effort are much discussed.

The way in which the original noble purpose needs to be refracted in the contemporary world and the manner in which both direct and indirect activities contribute to mission are deeply pondered. A constant return to mission as a motif central to discernment is emphasized. Formation programs expect leaders to be able to articulate mission concerns within the context of their own sphere of responsibility.

Organizational liturgy emerges. Leaders are expected to build reflection and prayer into meetings and organizational events, not just as bookends, but as integral parts of the actual processing of strategic decisions. They are expected to be able to symbolize the organization's ethos at punctuated moments in the flow of organizational life: at beginnings, when achieving important benchmarks, and in closings. They are expected to learn the language symbols of meaning that are part of the organization's tradition, and to value supportive rites and rituals that keep culture central in organizational life.

Their own style of leadership is expected to be congruent with organizational culture and to create within their own organizational unit an "oasis of goodness" where a holistic concern with individual dignity, inclusion in appropriate decision-making, rewards for normatively positive behavior, and sanctions for inappropriate behavior demonstrate that there is not a disconnect between espoused culture and daily realities. Leaders set the tone for relationships, decision processing, conflict resolution, and compassionate concern for each associate. Research shows that how an associate is supported in times of personal crises is the litmus test of cultural authenticity.

The culture arena is often seen as one of the success stories associated with leadership formation. Leaders who have completed formation programs seem more in tune with and supportive of the mission, values, and implicit culture of their sponsoring organizations.

Still there are stresses. Stewardship that requires increased efficiencies, change that requires radical readjustments, market shifts that require workforce dislocations, technology changes that displace prior skills, demographic shifts that make prior services obsolete, and many other difficult realities make maintaining culture a delicate matter. Working through such tough realities in a manner that is not destructive of culture takes spiritual presence and careful discernment. Failures such as the right decision made the wrong way without sufficient dialogue and inclusion, the right action carried out insensitively, the behavior of a key role player who acts immaturely, and a thousand other organizational viruses can mortally wound a culture for a period of time.

There is also the sensitive issue of religious pluralism. Organizations founded within a religious tradition such as health care or education no longer are staffed only by members of that tradition, nor are their clients only from their tradition. So there is a struggle to learn how to be true to the essential elements of a cultural tradition while at the same time being hospitable to and learning from other traditions. This antinomy is a long way from being resolved.

Closing

The purpose of this chapter has been to illustrate how leadership formation is different from but enriching of leadership development. Each has its own intellectual roots. Leadership development's roots are in the social, organizational, and management sciences. Leadership formation's roots are in religious and spiritual wisdom.

We can hardly choose between these important forms of leadership enrichment. To do so would be to subscribe to a false dualism that separates spirituality from organizational life. After a very secular half century, the mega-trend interest in spirituality attests that there is a need for both scientific and spiritual insight. Leadership formation brings spiritual understanding and practices to enrich the repertoire of critical competences modern leadership demands.

In the words of Parker Palmer,

> A leader is someone with the power to project either shadow or light onto some part of the world and onto the lives of the people who dwell there. A leader shapes the ethos in which others must live, an ethos as light-filled as heaven or as shadowy as hell. A good leader is intensely aware of the interplay of inner shadow and light, lest the act of leadership do more harm than good.[1]

Notes

1. Parker J. Palmer, *Let Your Life Speak: Listening for the Voice of Vocation* (San Francisco: Jossey-Bass, 2000), 78.

Practices

of the

Ministry Leadership
Formation Program

CHAPTER 5

Adaptive Challenges in the Ministry Leadership Formation Program

John Shea

As we implemented our leadership formation program, certain issues and situations became adaptive challenges.[1] They were recurring elements that had to be addressed and readdressed. Every way of developing and aligning them unfolded into further possibilities, changes that would make them better suited to reach their goals. We talk about these issues and situations in comparative language: "This is better than before, but it still needs work. How does this sync with that?" Often we intuit the need for greater refinement and focus before we find the right language to articulate this cutting edge. In short, these issues and situations are in need of continuous quality improvement.

A complete list of these issues and situations would become a recital of tedious details. But, in general, we have identified seven adaptive challenges: program content and sequence, presenters and staff, evaluation and measurement, off-site/on-site connections, adult learning method, system cooperation and collaboration, and alumni formation. This chapter describes the challenges involved in program content and sequence, presenters and staff, off-site/on-site connection, adult learning method, and alumni formation. Chapter 6 outlines how evaluation and measurement have accompanied and served the program, the participants, and the systems. Chapter 7 builds on this chapter's discussion of off-site/on-site possibilities by documenting the development of our website and the communication and community it makes possible for program participants, the sponsoring systems, and the larger public. Chapter 8 builds on this chapter's discussion of adult learning by identifying key aspects of facilitating and resourcing groups that result in effective formation. Chapter 9 explores the intersystem and intrasystem organizational context of the Ministry Leadership Program and connects it with the overall formation efforts within those systems.

Identifying these different adaptive challenges is helpful for educational and organizational purposes. But the challenges should never be separated. In the full experience of designing and implementing a formation program, they overlap and influence one another. For example, evaluation and measurement is an integral part of every challenge; alumni formation is crucial to the goals of system cooperation and collaboration; adult learning method is intimately connected to program content and sequence; and web technology and e-learning has made a game-changing impact on off-site/on-site connections and positively contributes to every challenge. The interconnected whole is always the context for focusing on specific parts.

> We identified seven adaptive challenges—program content and sequence, presenters and staff, evaluation and measurement, off-site/on-site connections, adult learning method, system cooperation and collaboration, and alumni formation.

In addition, as the name "adaptive challenge" indicates, each area has a history, a path of change and development. For example, how we inhabited and worked with off-site/on-site connections in 2006 is not how we did it in 2009; and how we did it 2009 has been considerably modified to meet what is happening in 2013. In our description of these areas, sometimes we chart this progression because it is crucial to understanding the substance of the challenge. Other times we describe the challenge as we presently formulate it without noting how or why it morphed into this particular formulation. But whether our description of a specific challenge includes the course of its development or not, the assumption is that evaluation and change was, is, and will be an essential component.

Program Content and Sequence

Chapter 2, "The Process and Content of Leadership Formation," outlined some of the issues in program content and sequence. There is the need to clarify the content of the Catholic ethos, to demarcate the distinctiveness of the Catholic identity and mission. We did this by identifying the twelve foundational concerns of the tradition: Vocation, Heritage, Spirituality, Responding to Suffering, Values Integration, Catholic Social Teaching, Discernment, Whole Person Care, Care for the Poor, Organizational Ethics, Clinical Ethics, and Collaboration with Church Authorities and Agencies.[2] But we also acknowledged the limits of just naming these concerns. Their specific content is still undetermined, and it cannot be established arbitrarily and presented in a standard educational format. It has to be shaped to the realities of health care in general and to the everyday activities of leaders in particular. A step in that direction was transposing the foundational concerns into an avowal statement

In short, these issues and situations are in need of continuous quality improvement.

of the identity and work of leaders in Catholic Health Care. For example, Values Integration is expressed: "As leaders of Catholic Health Care, we work to integrate core values into organizational structures, policies, and behaviors."

The key aid in this project of determining the relevant content of the foundational concerns is the Triangle. If the tradition's foundational concerns are put in dialogue with relevant cultural information and the individual and communal experience of the leaders, they can be fashioned into leadership tools. For example, when the concern of Vocation interfaces with the cultural information on the work attitudes of job, career, and calling, it becomes a way to assess co-worker morale. When the concern of Responding to Suffering interfaces with the cultural information on compassionate organizations, it highlights leadership challenges in dealing with the suffering of co-workers. When the concern of Discernment interfaces with the cultural information on strategic decision-making, it gives leaders a way to enhance one of their major responsibilities. Staying in the harness of the Triangle is the best way to ensure the connection between the distinctive concern and leadership responsibility.

> If the tradition's foundational concerns are put in dialogue with relevant cultural information and the individual and communal experience of the leaders, they can be fashioned into leadership tools.

Our formation program has been operational for seven years. During that time, using the Triangle, we have identified specific content for the twelve concerns that are relevant to Catholic Health Care and leadership activities. We have also fashioned adult learning procedures to communicate this content. As the introduction indicated, we are presently working on leadership workbooks and formers' guides for each of the twelve concerns. These books will spell out the specific content and processes of leadership formation.

However, as we worked with the Triangle, two questions repeatedly surfaced. The first question was, after the tradition sets the agenda by naming the foundational concerns, what else does it offer? The general answer is that it offers the theological considerations (including both scriptural and post-scriptural developments) and the ethical considerations of each foundational concern. *The Ethical and Religious Directives* (ERDs) of the National Conference of Catholic Bishops are the prime example. We include the ERDs within our twelve foundational concerns. In particular, they are incorporated into the concerns of Heritage, Spirituality, Catholic Social Teaching, Whole Person Care, Clinical Ethics, and Organizational Ethics. Since these theological and ethical perspectives are official positions and were crafted and re-crafted to respond to health care situations, they are directly applicable to leadership responsibilities. But to effectively express and communicate them, they are best positioned within these larger theological and ethical contexts.

The second question was, how do the concerns of the tradition actually interact with the information from the culture and individual and communal experience? In a model that stresses conversation between three sources, one of challenges is to make sure each source contributes. At certain times and under certain pressures, we are tempted to short-circuit the process. One of the three sources is not sufficiently consulted, and so there is not sufficient representation. However, even when there are three contributing voices, their interaction is not assured. There can be three monologues, each having an agenda so strong that it does not listen to the perspectives of the other sources. The result is three parallel speeches that never manage to become the valued conversation that will provide the fullest appreciation of situations and suggest the most effective action.[3]

The ideal unfolding of a Triangle conversation should be an orderly progression. In this ideal, tradition, having set the agenda, interacts with any cultural information that can inform the agenda. Once that is done, individual and communal experience evaluates what it has heard and makes decisions about what is relevant in leadership situations. However, actual processes of reflection seldom play by orderly rules. They may begin by expressing individual and communal experience, noting how the larger culture influences it, and then asking how the tradition affirms and critiques it. In other words, all three sources need to be included and all three sources need to interact with one another. But the conversation can start from any of the sources and proceed in a zigzag fashion. This adds complexity to the adaptive challenge: not only do the foundational concerns need to be turned into leadership tools through the use of the Triangle, the Triangle conversation needs to be conducted in different ways depending on the concern and the participants.[4]

The content of the foundational concerns is closely connected to the sequence of the concerns. Our program unfolds over three years, with four off-site sessions each year.[5] How should these sessions be sequenced, organized, and presented? Is knowledge of one of the concerns a necessary condition for understanding other concerns? Chapter 2, on the process and content of formation, described our temporal order as one year focusing on the identity of the Catholic Health Care leader and two years focusing on the work. The sequence in the first year is Vocation, Heritage, Spirituality, and Responding to Suffering and it always remains in that order.[6] The sequence for the next two years has varied, mainly because of presenter availability. Evaluations have suggested that Whole Person Care should be early in those two years, that Clinical and Organizational Ethics should be back to back, and that Collaboration with Church Authorities and Agencies should conclude the program. This basic distinction and connection between the identity and work of Catholic Health Care leaders provides a clear framework for the three years.

However, no matter how the sessions are sequenced, formation is a more complex and overlapping process than creating a logical order. In the minds of leaders, the sessions have their own interactive life. Leaders report getting "spirituality" when they are working with "whole person care." Or they come to understand the crucial importance of "heritage" when they are working with "care for the poor." Or, they remark that "it came together after the fifth session," but without mentioning the content of the fifth session. Identity and work are mutually reinforcing; and their temporal sequence in the program is not as significant as how and when they connect and have an impact on each other in the minds and actions of the leaders. This is part of the mystery of attraction developed in chapter 2 and that is crucial to socialization into the community and tradition.

Presenters and Staff

The staff of the Ministry Leadership Center presents the first two sessions of the program.[7] The first session includes a half-day of introductory material and a day-and-a-half on the foundational concern of Vocation. The second session concentrates on Heritage. However, a co-agenda of these two sessions is community building. The participants get to know one another and the staff gets to know the participants. This happens through formal group processes as well as at meals, social hours, and free time. Communal relations are a key factor in the learning dynamics of the program, and it has to be explicitly attended to from the beginning.

At these opening sessions the role of the staff is both to present the foundational concerns of Vocation and Heritage and to provide hospitality and service to the gathered leaders. Hospitality and service cannot be underestimated. Staff members are present at the door to welcome participants as they arrive, and they stand at the door wishing them safe travels as they leave. The guiding principle is that it begins before it begins and it continues after its over. Formation is not program-centered. It is centered on people who are engaging a program to develop themselves as leaders. In addition, between arrival and departure, any concerns of the participants are immediately dealt with. At the beginning of every session the executive director reminds them that the Ministry Leadership Center staff will help them with anything that comes up; and many things do come up—a broken showerhead, an emergency call from home or work, printing boarding passes, special dietary requests, a cushion for a bad back, and so on.

The staff will accompany the participants through all twelve sessions. Each session is a day and a half. On the first day, a visiting presenter leads the group into the foundational concern; and on the second morning the staff processes the first day and presents more input/exercises on the foundational concern. The staff provides continuity in the program, gets to know the leaders and their particular learning paths, and creates a community atmosphere. The overall atmosphere is relaxed and dress is informal. It is a gathering of concerned people who are reflecting on their leadership in light of the foundational concerns of their organizational culture. In short, the staff walks with the leaders through their three-year formation program, ensuring a friendly and open tone to the sessions.

> Hospitality and service cannot be underestimated. Staff members are present at the door to welcome participants as they arrive and they stand at the door wishing them safe travels as they leave.

On the first day for nine of the sessions, there is a visiting presenter. Although we have had excellent presenters from within the six systems that we serve, we usually draw from outside the systems for the sake of variety and newness. We work with presenters beforehand to make sure they will fit into the program. We send them material, discuss what they intend to present and how they intend to present it, determine what the pre-session requirements will be, design an evaluation tool for their session, and so on. (See appendix A and appendix B.) If we do not work extensively with presenters, they will most likely give canned lectures that will not be sufficiently shaped to the experience and responsibility of our leaders.

But we also have to work with the participants about how to relate to the presenters. We see the presenters as resource people for the concerns and issues of leaders and not teachers of a topic that leaders have to learn. This is a subtle distinction, but it entails an important attitude both on the part of the participants and on the part of the presenters. The participants are not expected to enter the world of the presenters and struggle with their concerns. They are expected to assess what the presenters have to offer them and to make sure they get from the presenters what they want and need. In other words, they have to become active in their own learning.

We see the presenters as resource people for the concerns and issues of leaders and not teachers of a topic that leaders have to learn.

In turn, the presenters are not expected to say everything they know in a given area or to import academic agendas into their presentations. They are expected to know and find the opening in leadership experience for the knowledge they possess and to present that knowledge in a way that connects with that opening. In short, they are encouraged to creatively interact and not just to talk. A practical implication of this idea of presenters as resource people is the length of their presentation. We suggest keeping any presentation under thirty minutes and connecting it with a table exercise. If participants understand that they are interacting with a resource person and if presenters understand that they are primarily resources, their interaction with each other will be mutually beneficial.

With the six groups who have been through the program or are presently in the program, we have had the same presenters for three of the sessions and we have had turnovers in seven of the sessions. The stability is because the presenters are excellent and fit in with the culture of the program. They and we work well together. The turnovers were for various reasons. Some reasons were simply logistical, like scheduling conflicts and unavailability.

Other reasons were because of program changes. The staff decided to go another way with a particular session and a different presenter was needed. Other reasons were because presenters were too abstract, or lacked adult learning skills, or did not make a sufficient enough effort to fit in with the goals and culture of the program.

In the MLC formation program, the staff accompanies the leaders through the three years. We recruit and vet the best presenters to enter into this process and catalyze it with their knowledge and experience. But, as important as presenters are, we are not a presenter-driven or a presenter-dependent program. When a presenter does an excellent job (and that is 98 percent of the time), the staff builds on that and helps the leaders internalize the learning and integrate it into their work. When a presenter misses the mark, the staff uses that miss to help the leaders identify what the true target is and how they can hit it themselves. We believe that the best way to think about formation is to see it as staff and leaders using resource people (the presenters) to facilitate and achieve their goals.

Off-Site/On-Site Connections

The most challenging area for our program, and we suspect for all leadership programs, is maintaining the connection between what is done off-site at our sessions and what happens when the leaders return to their work situations, their on-site leadership activities.[8] The geographical and cultural dynamics are:

- moving from a work situation in an organization to a reflective situation in a retreat house;

- acquiring the working knowledge and skills of the organization's foundational concerns in the retreat house; and

- returning to the work situation and shaping it according to the knowledge and skills initially acquired in the retreat house.

The challenge underneath these travel arrangements and cultural shifts has to be honored.

This challenge is basically to determine what can happen during the three months between sessions. If there is not some ongoing formation activity during that time, the sessions will be a series of interruptions from work. Formation will only come on the leaders' radar four times a year: "Oh, it's time to head out to MLC again" is all they will think. A key component of this challenge is to determine what the leaders are doing with what they have learned. Since the purpose of leadership formation is organizational transformation, leaders have to articulate and integrate what they are learning into their work situations. We initially named this expectation "teaching" and later changed it to "Action|Feedback." Leaders are expected to engage their co-workers in some type of action that would integrate the foundational concern into their organization. However, it is one thing to have this as a program expectation, but it is quite another thing to be able to supply the interpersonal support and structural accountability for this expectation to be met.

We have gone through two phrases with this adaptive challenge of connecting off-site sessions with on-site situations. In the first phrase, we put in place four on-site expectations: tracking ideas, reading and reflecting, dialogue partners, and teaching. Each of the six systems adapted these expectations to suit their culture and modus operandi. (See appendix C.) These four expectations were spelled out in the following way:

1. Tracking Ideas: Between off-site sessions the participants will track ideas that continue the learnings of the previous sessions. These ideas will be triggered by general work experiences,

by reading and reflecting on monthly one-page papers that arrive via email, and by gathering the learnings from the conversations with the dialogue partner and the teaching experience. This tracking may take the form of ongoing journaling, or jotting notes that summarize key ideas, or writing a paragraph or two that captures an idea and its implications. Some written form is essential to fulfilling the expectation of tracking ideas.

2. Reading and Reflecting: In the middle of the months when there is no off-site session, one-page papers that develop the learnings of the off-site sessions will arrive via email. They will include reflection questions. Participants will read and reflect on these papers, journaling the answers to the questions. (See appendix D.)

3. Dialoging with a Partner: Each participant will have a dialogue partner. The participant will meet with his or her partner once a month. In general, the conversation should be anywhere between a half hour and an hour. The purpose of the conversation is greater clarity in how the participants are thinking and greater relevance to what they do. To facilitate this conversation, the dialogue partner will receive a one-page summary of what the previous off-site session covered. (See appendix E.)

4. Teaching: Participants will lead their management teams in a fifteen- to thirty-minute exercise that focuses on the learnings of the off-site sessions. These exercises and instructions on how to facilitate them will be given during the off-site session. Where two or more participants are members of the same leadership team, they may choose to work together on a single exercise.

As the program progressed, it became clear that these expectations did not carry equal weight. Tracking ideas, especially in written form, usually fell by the wayside. The one-page reflection papers went out monthly, and there was occasional feedback. Informal surveys suggested that about half of the participants spent some time with them, and that many used them with their dialogue partners. However, it was the dialogue partners and the teaching that became the chief carriers of formation between the off-site sessions.

Although the dialogue partners were supported and coordinated by the systems, many practical problems made persevering in monthly meetings difficult. But for those who managed to stay with a dialogue partner, it became an important formation relationship. A survey summary found dialogue partners very valuable but difficult to prioritize. Its value was that participants found a colleague to debrief with, a safe harbor to express their thoughts and feelings. Some of the leaders developed deep relationships with their dialogue partners that continued long after the program was completed. In addition, as the number of leaders who had been through the program grew into a critical mass within the systems and at individual sites, in some places— corporate and regional offices and specific facilities—dialogue partners morphed into dialogue groups. From the staff point of view, dialogue partners kept formation ideas and behaviors in mind between sessions and contributed to the skills of articulation and integration.

> Some of the leaders developed deep relationships with their dialogue partners that continued long after the program was completed.

We gave most attention to the teaching expectation. This represented the critical movement from leader formation to organizational transformation. From the beginning, a concern was that the program would turn into a three-year leadership renewal experience. The leaders themselves would be refreshed and energized, but the organization would not be affected. Although it could be argued that if leaders came to know and understand the identity and mission of Catholic Health Care in a more complete and relevant way, the knowledge would naturally overflow into their leadership responsibilities, that surmise was leaving too much to chance. There had to be structural support and accountability. Otherwise, in the busy and hectic days of health care executives, formation ideas and behaviors would not be included.

Our first attempt to supply this support and accountability was to bookend the workplace possibility. For example, at the session on Values Integration, leaders would plan their workplace teaching and share those plans with one another (for a half hour). At the next session, there was an informal debriefing where participants reported on what they had done and the feedback they received (for one hour). However, between the sessions there did not seem to be any realistic way to provide support or accountability. After all, in any given group there were 120 participants spread through six systems in twelve states. The development of the MLC website brought new possibilities and a second phrase began.

In the second phrase of connecting off-site and on-site experiences, we recognized that "teaching" was too narrow a word for the range of leadership opportunities that were available for integrating the foundational concerns. We changed the on-site expectation to "Action|Feedback." At the same time, we brought a better balance to how we broke out the six systems at the sessions. We had always mixed them, even when they were planning and reporting on their on-site activities. Now we kept people in their own systems for both planning and reporting.

> There had to be structural support and accountability. Otherwise, in the busy and hectic days of health care executives, formation ideas and behaviors would not be included.

This meant we developed system "forums" within each cohort who would supply support and accountability both within the sessions and between the sessions. It was the website and the introduction of blended learning that made this all possible. This development will be detailed in chapter 7, "Formation, Technology, and Blended Learning."

Adult Learning Method

There are many statements of the principles of adult learning in general and how they might be applied to different situations, especially leadership activities.[9] Multiple models describe the steps of highly motivated people in their efforts to learn skills that will make them more effective in specific settings.[10] There are established techniques like identifying optimal learning styles, seeking data-based feedback, enlisting coaches, detailing specific skills, and engaging tools for self-evaluation and behavior measurement. But only leaders who have a desire to engage in personal and professional development profit from these methods of adult learning.[11]

At MLC, we situate adult learning method within the Triangle. In the Triangle, individual and communal experience evaluates the agenda that has been developed from the dialogue between tradition and cultural information.[12]

This evaluative action presupposes that leaders have been engaged in the present; and this present engagement is driving them to evaluate past experience and consider how their future experience should be shaped. Adult learning method is about present engagement that evaluates past experience and directs future experience. The initial task of our program is to catalyze this development process by forceful engagement in the present.

> Only leaders who have a desire to engage in personal and professional development profit from these methods of adult learning.

From the beginning of the program, we knew that engaging experience—present, past, and future—was the key to effective formation. But our ability to do it was not as developed as our conviction that it was necessary. Gradually, we improved. For example, before every session we send out pre-session material. At first, we would just send out a reading on the foundational concern. Then we began to attach instructions on how to read the reading and what to look for as well as questions to answer upon completing the reading. We hoped this would help engagement. At first, many of the readings would remain in the background. We would not refer to them at the sessions. Then, we began to work with each reading during the sessions. Now, everything that is done pre-session is worked with in-session. This increases the motivation to do the pre-session work.

To further encourage engagement, we added interviews and input/exercises to the pre-session work. For example, the pre-session work for Responding to Suffering includes the following task: "Please contact a chaplain or spiritual caregiver and interview them using the question: 'What have you learned about suffering that everyone in the organization should know?' Capture their response and be prepared to express and communicate it during our session on Responding to Suffering."

Input/exercises are different from readings. They are short perspectives—two or three pages—on some aspect of the foundational concern accompanied by an exercise that connects the input to the participant's experience. (See appendix F.) Both these modifications—interviews and input/exercises—have increased leader engagement in the foundational concern.

These are some of the ways that we have tried to elicit the source of individual and communal experience and bring it into the Triangle conversation in one aspect of our program—pre-session requirements. But we carry the agenda of increased engagement into every aspect of the program. It would be too detailed to survey the many forms this agenda takes—case studies, model practices, and so on. But there are three techniques that are repeatedly used to ensure a relevant connection of the foundational concerns to the experience of the leaders.

The first falls into the general category of assessment tool. Every presentation or input has to produce a way of surfacing and analyzing an area of experience that leaders can use to examine their own experience of that area. In different words, it has to develop a model to look through and see something that is already there but may have escaped notice. For example, in the concern of Whole Person Care, a model of support and burnout is presented and then used by leaders to assess their own experience of support and burnout. Once the model allows an area of experience to be seen and assessed, the "burden of knowing" unfolds into the "call to action." The leaders have to determine how to respond to what they now see. In this way, all three temporal dimensions are happening. The strength of the present engagement is urging an evaluation of the past and a proposal for the future.

The second technique overlaps with the first and falls into the general category of reflection on experience. What type of experience is retrieved is determined by the tradition that sets the agenda. This retrieval process begins by formulating a recall question beginning with "recall a time when" or some equivalent phrasing. For example, in the Responding to Suffering session, leaders are asked to "recall a time within the organization when you were treated compassionately. What were the features of that compassionate treatment?" However, the skill of this technique is not only the ability to remember. It is ability to express the remembered experience in story form, and then to distill that story into conceptual language. The leaders who are able to express their experience in both narrative and concept make the foundational concerns come alive. In this way, they increase the engagement of the entire group with the foundational concern.

The third technique is much more than a technique. It is the practice of silence, recommended by all religious traditions and many psychological traditions. We begin the first and second days of our off-site sessions with three to five minutes of silence. We characterize silence as a house with many rooms. In each room there are instructions about what to do with the silence. (See appendix G.) We give instructions to the participants about a possible use for the silent time.[13] The instructions usually match the foundational concern the leaders will be engaging during the session. But we always encourage the leaders to use the silence in a way that seems right to them on this particular day at this particular moment. The practice of silence increases their ability and desire for interiority. Interiority is a key factor in the formation process.

For us, learning takes place when individuals are set within a community of co-learners with a key person who is directing that learning. We recognize that learning is an individual affair. People will develop in their own way, both at a different pace and at a different depth. But in our program, from beginning to end, we situate individual growth within communal and professional support and encouragement. Within the day-and-a-half off-site session, the leaders are interacting with one another and with a person who is directing the interaction. In their time between sessions, they are in contact with one another through dialogue partners and website interaction.

> For us, learning takes place when individuals are set within a community of co-learners and a key person who is directing that learning.

For the most part, we work on the assumption that individual development flourishes within community relationships.

A key actor in this communal learning is the person directing it. The traditional name for this person is "teacher." But we have not been satisfied with the title "teacher." Although it is the traditional name, it also carries the connotation of someone who has all the knowledge and tries to tell it to others—the infamous from jug to mug approach. Also, the word instantly triggers memories. It taps into previous educational experiences. Some leaders have had very good educational experiences and some have had very bad educational experiences. But, whether good or bad, most have had passive educational experience. They listen to teachers, privately evaluate them, and go their way. The connection between entertainment and education is very prominent.

Therefore, we have experimented with different ways of naming the role of the person directing the learning process. They are "presenters" because they bring forward knowledge of the tradition and the culture. But they are also "facilitators" because they have to connect this knowledge with leadership situations, and that entails helping leaders articulate their experience. Sometimes we just call them "formers" because what we are about is the work of formation that socializes individuals into a community/tradition. But when we looked carefully at how we think maximal learning occurs, we identified those directing the process as facilitator/resource people.

Their primary task is to make learning happen in communal settings whose dynamics quickly change, blocking some paths of advance and opening others. This entails a variety of skills that have to come together as an artful activity that discerns the shifting possibilities. But more than facilitation skills are needed. At times, the learning process has to be resourced. Knowledge has to be inserted—sometimes to have a settling effect and sometimes to have a stirring effect. This means not only having knowledge but also being able to call upon that knowledge to resource the conversation. These dynamics of facilitation/resource, which are crucial to formational learning, will be elaborated in more detail in the chapter "Facilitation/Resource in Leadership Formation."

Alumni Formation

The majority of leaders who complete the program express a strong desire to continue formation. At the present moment, MLC provides four resources to assist this continuing formation. The first is a series of videos and podcasts that are formatted for individual or group use. These resources are on significant leadership qualities: "The Ethical Leader," "The Prophetic Leader," "The Reflective Leader," "The Listening Leader," and "The Integral Leader." They can be downloaded from the MLC website.

The second resource is reunion cohorts. These are day-and-a-half formation sessions on significant topics. We have met with national leaders in health care to discuss "The Catholic Health Care Ministry and Church Relations: Natural Tensions"; "Health Care Reform: The Catholic Leadership Response"; "Spirituality and Leadership: Empirical Data, Qualitative Analysis, and Theological Reflection"; and "Workforce Reductions: Spiritual and Organizational Responses." These programs are scheduled to allow for broad participation and arranged to permit leaders to attend all or part of the program and still derive substantial benefit.

The third resource is a pilot program, the senior leadership cohort. Laurence O'Connell, Diarmuid Rooney, and Andre Delbecq have convened, facilitated, and resourced this effort. Andre Delbecq wrote this description:

The senior leadership cohort is a pilot program paralleling leadership development groups such as the Young Presidents Organization or Vistage. In these very effective programs a group of senior leaders gather regularly to reflect and dialogue together regarding timely leadership topics (e.g., personal challenges such as managing stress and overload, or organizational challenges such as strategic positioning). In the second part of the gathering, individual leaders share difficult personal challenges. Examples might be a vexing reporting relationship, or uncertainty regarding how to process a forthcoming critical meeting with conflictive stakeholders. Over time each leader benefits from the pooled judgments of their colleagues, acquiring new skills and information, and learning street-smart ways of proceeding—all the while being supported by a cohesive circle of trust while working through the challenge. Further, accountability comes into play since serious challenges are seldom resolved in one action, so one is accompanied over the duration of the challenge and are likely to report on actions taken and lessons learned leading to double-loop learning.

The senior leadership cohort adds spiritual overlays. Short spiritual passages are provided for spiritual reflection relating to the theme of a meeting. Periods of meditative silence punctuate periods of dialogue. Spiritual insights from the earlier leadership formation program are referenced and readings are provided so that theological insight is aligned with best leadership practices. Judgments are pooled in the spirit of discernment including careful attention to mission and values. Spiritual practices are engaged so that the sharing goes beyond rational, analytic decision-making. A leader and all those feel the impact of a reported challenge are held in prayer.

As this cycle repeats itself over time, the manner of how a spiritually mature leader proceeds to process complex decisions is learned through the sharing of lived experiences.

Preliminary evaluation suggests that the senior leadership cohort is valued for providing a small circle of trust where difficult leadership problems can be sifted and winnowed in a non-judgmental environment. The cohort is seen as a place where the leader's "whole person" is touched and supported. The cohort is valued as a setting in which the challenges of developing greater spiritual and psychological maturity become visible. But above all, the cohort is seen as a source of support exactly when the leader is most vulnerable, when wrestling with seemingly intractable problems.

The senior leadership cohort pilot program is providing valuable insights into how more localized ongoing formation could be conducted.

The fourth resource is the international cohort. In 2010 the first international cohort of participants were invited to travel to Constantinople and Asia Minor (modern-day Turkey), where much of the early Christian tradition took shape, as well as critical turning points in the development of the Jewish and Islamic traditions. A second cohort is being planned for the summer of 2013.

Conclusion

By the time this book is in print, each of these adaptive challenges, as their name implies, will have adapted. Program content and sequence will have been further refined, the various roles of the staff and presenters will have been sharpened, and alumni formation will have been developed along a number of paths that the alumni, MLC, and the sponsoring systems determine. But, at this stage, the four challenges that are undergoing significant development are how we do evaluation and measurement, how we use technology and blended learning to hold together off-site and on-site experiences, how we facilitate adult learning, and how we interact with the sponsoring systems and how they cooperate and collaborate with one another. The next four chapters will elaborate how these challenges are being addressed.

Notes

1. "Adaptive challenge" is a phrase associated with Ronald Heifetz, Donald Laurie, and Marty Linsky. See Heifetz and Laurie, "The Work of Leadership," *Harvard Business Review*, January-February, 1997; and Heifetz and Linsky, *Leadership on the Line: Staying Alive through the Dangers of Leading* (Cambridge, Mass.: Harvard Business Review Press, 2002). They connect it to the leadership challenge of being able to distinguish situations that are problems to be solved from situations that are ongoing challenges to which the people most affected by them have to continually adapt. We use "adaptive challenge" in a relaed but different way. The phrase signals the "continuous quality improvement" approach that is necessary in formation programing.

2. Early in our program, we had an ongoing conversation around what is Catholic about Catholic Health Care. Since Catholic Health Care participates in U.S. health care and, in most ways, conforms to the requirements and standards of this larger reality, it can look like just one more instance of health care in America. As one participant said of Catholic Health Care, "Nothing different really."

At first the conversation was framed as, "What makes Catholic Health Care unique?" Implicit in this framing was a marketing perspective. Was there something about Catholic Health Care that gave it a marketing advantage? If there was, could it be named and used? But this uniqueness framing gave way to the question of distinctiveness: "What makes Catholic Health Care distinctive?" Uniqueness denotes that no one else has this quality. Distinctiveness denotes that others may have this quality, but that it also is a major concern of Catholic Health Care; when it is put in concert with other qualities, it results in a distinctive way of being a health care organization. Implicit in this framing is an organizational identity and mission perspective.

3. Chapter 3, "Ministry Leadership Formation: Theological Grounding and Method," is an example of dialogue between perspectives from the tradition and cultural wisdom about areas of leadership activity.

4. Chapter 3, "Ministry Leadership Formation: Theological Grounding and Method," goes into more detail about Triangle conversations.

5. Formation is different. Absorbing values and purpose into the fabric of one's life and learning to lead from a well-integrated mission is an ongoing process, entailing difficult inner work. It evolves slowly, with the initial phase lasting many months, if not years. The extended time is an acknowledgment that formation involves much more than acquiring a body of information. John O. Mudd, "When Knowledge and Skills Aren't Enough," *Health Progress*, September-October, 2009.

6. There have been two times when presenter availability forced us to put the Responding to Suffering session before the Spirituality session.

7. Laurence J. O'Connell, John Shea, Diarmuid Rooney, Elizabeth McCabe, Mary Anne Sladich-Lantz, Sharyn Lee, and Catherine Alesci.

8. For a different view of on this complex dynamic of off-site/on-site formation, see John Glaser and Deborah A. Proctor, "Keeping Formation In House Deepens Catholic Culture," *Health Progress*, September-October, 2011.

9. For a general overview of adult learning methods, see Sharan B. Merriam, Rosemary S. Caffarella, and Lisa M. Baumgartner, *Learning in Adulthood: A Comprehensive Guide*, 3rd ed. (San Francisco: Jossey-Bass, 2007). For adult learning methods applied to leadership development, see Ellen van Velsor, Cynthia D. McCauley, and Marian N. Ruderman, *The Center for Creative Leadership Handbook of Leadership Development*, 3rd ed. (San Francisco: Jossey-Bass, 2010).

10. See, e.g., Richard Boyatzis and Annie McKee, *Resonant Leadership* (Cambridge, Mass.: Harvard Business School Press, 2005), chap. 5, "Intentional Change."

11. An initial guide to the area of personal development is Michael Waters, *The Element Dictionary of Personal Development* (Rockport, Md.: Element Books, 1996).

12. See chapter 3, "Ministry Leadership Formation: Theological Grounding and Method," for a more developed interpretation of the Triangle and adult learning.

13. In the Spirituality session, the presenter uses silence to give instructions on centering prayer and leads participants in this spiritual practice.

CHAPTER 6

Evaluation and Measurement in Leadership Formation

William McCready

One of the great mistakes is to judge policies and programs by their intentions rather than their results.

— Milton Friedman

The purpose of evaluation is to create greater understanding of a particular program or activity through documenting improvement and accountability. In the Leadership Formation Program of the Ministry Leadership Center this means (a) understanding how each session has an impact on individual participants, and (b) how participation both by individuals and through the additive influence of multiple individuals leads to having an impact on participating health care institutions and systems. There is an evaluation paradox of trying to measure "spiritual" impact when "Spirit" moves outside the senses. We believe that the outcomes are not simply a matter of concept or self-practice, but also mediated by Spirit. Thus at the material level $1+1+1$ totals 3; but the Spirit may act within individuals or groups so that $1+1+1$ totals a greater sum. We of course cannot directly measure "Spirit," but since human nature is of body, mind, heart, and spirit, the outcome of Spirit is manifested phenomenologically, and thus nuances of spiritual maturity are sensed both within and by others. We "know" when we are in the presence of an integrated (whole or holy) person who is spiritually mature, and we "know" when we are in the presence of a broken narcissist. Thus, in our measurement of outcomes we recognize up front that results reflect not only the learning materials, concepts, and practices contained within the program design, but are also impacted by the movement of Spirit.

This chapter describes four elements of the evaluation practice we have initiated at MLC: (1) using theoretical models to guide data collection and analyses; (2) measuring individual formation outcomes at both the session and end-of-formal-program levels; (3) assessing system-level formation outcomes with pilot studies; and (4) designing and implementing a Leadership Assessment Tool based on the twelve foundational concerns that are the core of the MLC program.

Using Theoretical Models to Guide Data Collection and Analyses

The MLC evaluation plan combines elements of program evaluation with the measurement of the outcomes of adult learning and the adoption of innovations. Everett Rogers formalized the theory about how innovations are adopted in a book called *Diffusion of Innovations*, published in 1962.[1] Rogers stated that adopters of any new innovation or idea could be generally categorized as one of these types:

- innovators (2.5 percent), who tend to be risk-takers;

- early adopters (13.5 percent), who tend to be sociable leaders;

- early majority (34 percent), who tend to have many social contacts;

- late majority (34 percent), who tend to be initial skeptics favoring the status quo; and

- laggards (16 percent), who tend to defer to friends' responses.

This distribution is based on a bell curve, and each adopter's willingness and ability to adopt an innovation depends on a variety of personal and situational characteristics. Formation is comparable to the adoption of innovations because it consists of a person learning new skills and then practicing them in day-to-day activities. Rogers also proposed a five-stage model to describe the diffusion of innovation that dovetails nicely with our model of adult learning and formation. The stages of diffusion are:

1. knowledge: learning about the existence and function of the innovation;

2. persuasion: becoming convinced of the value of the innovation;

3. decision: committing to the adoption of the innovation;

4. implementation: putting the innovation to use;

5. confirmation: the ultimate acceptance (or rejection) of the innovation.

A model that generally describes the traditional arc of formation, which has been established by many religious orders, moves from the person perceiving that they have been called to the life, through living in a community under a rule, to acquiring a vision of how life is to be lived. Leaders usually emerge from this process via a communal vetting process. The traditional formation process starts with a call to the religious life. Then a community of like-minded people comes together to share a vision. They live under a "rule" that nurtures and focuses the call, and they share a view of how the vision makes a difference in the world. People attain positions of leadership via a community vetting process. (See figure 6.1.)

The evaluation is based on the measurement theory of Everett Rogers's Diffusion of Innovations.

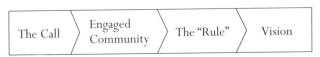

Figure 6.1 Traditional formation model

A model that describes the MLC formation process is a variation that follows a different arc. It moves from membership in a community (such as a hospital staff), through the formation program, to acquiring a vision of life and profession, to perceiving a sense of call or vocation. This process creates a "community of colleagues" for an intense three-year period during which they share experiences through "a process of stories" and acquire a shared vision of health care in the world. This experience stimulates a "calling" that changes "occupation" into "vocation." People attain leadership via a collegial vetting process. (See figure 6.2.)

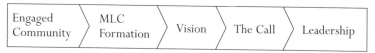

Figure 6.2 MLC formation model

The main difference between these models is the comparative role of "the rule" and the "MLC off-site program." In the traditional model the rule produces commitment to the community, and in the MLC model the three-year program, where each cohort stays together and shares experiences together, produces commitment to a vision. In both models articulating "stories" communicates the vision. The stories provide the glue that engenders community in the contemporary model similar to that forged in the traditional model by communal living.

Measuring Individual Formation Outcomes at Both the Session and End-of-Formal-Program Levels

This element of the evaluation focuses on two aspects of the program: (a) the improvement of the content, presentation, and dynamics of the twelve sessions; and (b) an assessment of what has been learned and applied over the three years of the formal program. To these ends we employed both quantitative surveys and qualitative reports from participants. There are three goals for the assessment aspect of the evaluation. The first is to measure the participants' abilities to articulate, reflect, and apply the insights they have acquired. The second is to detect and measure formational changes that can be defined as behaviors linked to the twelve foundational concerns at the program's core. The third is to measure participants' abilities to articulate and execute a vision of leadership in accord with those foundational concerns. To fulfill these goals, we conduct both pre- and post-session surveys and an assessment at the end of the three years. Both of these use qualitative and quantitative measures. Methodologists recommend this dual approach when studying outcomes that have multiple goals.

> We employed both quantitative surveys and qualitative reports from participants.

During the first years of the program, from 2005 through 2009, we conducted regular pre- and post-session surveys to find out what worked and what did not. These surveys ask questions about the relevance of session content to practical health care practices, about preferred styles of presentation, about what is learned and what needs to be learned, about interaction, and about the schedule and amenities. The usual survey format is to use ten-item, self-anchoring scales (to avoid the "midpoint dilemma," which stems from respondents' proclivity to over-select the middle of a scale) where only the two ends of the scale are labeled. For example, the labels may read "Not At All Helpful" and "Very Helpful," and the participants will use the ten points as they wish. The advantage of this technique is that respondents will choose their own way of using the scale (which is also why it is called "self-anchoring"). Some may use all ten points and others may use only the upper or lower half. Some may only use the middle of the scale and some may only use the poles. This allows for both aggregated and individual analysis of the responses.

We can estimate overall reaction by totaling the responses using all ten points across all respondents to get a summary measure on a particular program element, or we can standardize the scales for each individual's response pattern to produce measures that are independent of individual variations. This allows for a variety of analyses. We can explore sessions over time for consistency and the effects of innovation. We can explore sessions as they are experienced by successive groups of participants. We can also explore how individuals experience the program and develop their formation over time.

We conduct pre- and post-session surveys for the first three or four sessions as a way of establishing baselines against which to measure formational growth. (Initially we also used this technique to hone the program content.) Now, with the advent of the Leadership Assessment Tool, which will be discussed later in this chapter, we will be using a version of this tool to establish these baseline measures.

In addition to the session evaluations, we have used a variety of mechanisms to ask participants to recall significant things they have learned over the entire three years and the effects thereof. We also ask for reflections, which provides participants an unstructured opportunity to articulate their significant experiences in the program. Examples of typical summary findings from these "after three years" evaluations are:

- 88 percent wanted ongoing formation;
- 87 percent linked their formation with leadership;
- 81 percent were more open to religious pluralism;
- 79 percent acquired theological underpinnings;
- 77 percent had formed a community of leaders;
- 59 percent said the program had an effect in their system; and
- 46 percent said they were more confident in dealing with ethical tensions.

Summary themes that emerged from the qualitative analysis of the participants' reflections are:

- the experience of collegiality, learning from one another (92 percent mentioned);
- the importance of stories in articulating the vision (82 percent mentioned);
- the feeling that that the "vision changed how we work" (73 percent mentioned);
- the expression that they were "converted to formation" (51 percent mentioned);
- an improved understanding of ethics and decisions in the workplace (44 percent mentioned);
- the view that executives are "servant-leaders" (38 percent mentioned);
- the experience of a personal transformation (29 percent mentioned).

Evaluating the program begins with assessing the impact of each of the twelve day-and-a-half off-site sessions. Participants are asked to assess the contribution that the different sections (e.g., "The section on making connections between principles and organizational situations") of the off-site sessions (e.g., "Catholic Social Teaching") made to their working knowledge and skills. In this way they rate the program as to how it has affected them. This ongoing evaluation both measures the effectiveness of the individual program segments and provides the program designers with feedback, which is used to improve the program. The participants are also asked to reflect and articulate their own sense of having received working knowledge and skills that enhanced their abilities to lead the mission and ministry.

Personal growth, acquisition of theological underpinnings, and the bonding to a community of leaders are all products of the program.

Here are several examples of competencies that a majority of participants said they developed through their participation in the program. Of course, there are many other competencies that are being reported as part of the ongoing evaluation; this is only a sample. It is important to hear these competencies discussed in the words of the participants because articulation, along with integration, is a signal of the developing formation. (We have annotated the participants' comments to provide a context for understanding them better.) In discussing one competency, more than four-fifths mentioned that they connected *personal growth* with their development as leaders:

> *I have been changed by my experience of the MLC. . . . It is helpful for me not only in my calling [as a leader of Catholic Health Care], but also in my relationships, my physical life, and my intellectual life.*

> *As I reflect over the past three years, it is amazing how this changed my life—both personally and professionally. I am now more grounded in the theology and more able to share what I have learned with others. Yet, I am also very aware that to take care of others, I must also take time to care for myself and nurture my inner circle [of support].*

> *The greatest take away was making progress on my own spiritual journey.*

> *The MLC program has given me a stronger foundation to understand what it means to grow personally and professionally.*

Almost four-fifths mentioned they that they had *acquired theological underpinnings* critical to leadership:

> *I found the concept of "contrast experiences" to be very useful in getting to the deeper theological underpinnings of today's issues around suffering/wealth and insured/uninsured.*

> *Dignity, compassion, inclusion, and focusing on the greater good are values and perspectives which will provide valuable assistance*

when faced with difficult future challenges. I have always thought that the patient comes first, and now I know many more reasons why.

The foundational piece for me was the dignity of the human person. Where does it come from? When you strip away knowledge, money, position, appearance, friendships, family . . . do you still have human dignity? And the answer is yes, that our dignity comes to us as children of God. . . . Well this is also a bigger picture and contexts my work in even more meaningful ways.

Just over three-quarters mentioned that they embraced a community of Catholic Health Care leaders:

My work in Catholic Health Care allows me to connect my searching with the searching of other people . . . [to connect] with like-minded people who hold similar values . . . [and] to live those values along with [these] like-minded people.

I believe I have a strong inner circle of support. Throughout the past several years of leadership changes, our executive team has been modified. Since the last session, I have made a concerted effort to enhance the circles of support with my peers. This will allow for mutual support within our ministry. All of us will benefit from this effort. As our work environment is quite busy and geographically diverse, it is easy to operate within your own area. These walls and barriers need to be removed. This has been received well.

The shared and lived experience has indeed morphed the program into a community experience. These five systems have many aspects that are similar in their cultures, but live these values true, each to itself. It brought collective learning to a common experience which will have longer term opportunities to share. We have met others who now share a common language and common insights who can be mentors within their own organizations as well as across organizations.

As leaders analyze complex situations and fashion strategies to address them, they consult the mission and values that in
Catholic Health Care are theologically grounded. However, this
theological grounding is often bracketed or articulated in one or
two sentences—a "thin" description.[2] The result is that leaders
are not sure about underpinnings, do not know the convincing
rationales for certain positions, cannot make the link or follow
the logic, and are not fully aware of the bigger picture. However,
they want to know these theological underpinnings. Leaders strive
for knowledge. They want to be able to identify and articulate the
driving forces that influence the organization. This includes the
ultimate motivations, rationales, and perspectives of the faith-based
heritage. Therefore, they are appreciative when they acquire the
theological "whys" and are able to put it together with the critical
"whats" and the practical "hows."

This summary evaluation elicits (1) personal articulation and
reflection of their own leadership development, (2) their assessment of how their program cohort colleagues (from their own
systems) supported their growth and learned from one another,
and (3) observations of how what they and their colleagues have
learned in the program is becoming expressed within the practices
of the system. This reflects the adaptation of the traditional model
of formation. In the traditional model the "rule" produces commitment to the community, and in the MLC model the three years
of shared experiences produces collegiality and commitment to
a common vision. Shared and exchanged stories provide the glue
that binds the group together.

The year-three evaluation moves the focus from *how much* of
a contribution to *what* the contribution was. The final evaluation
seeks to understand the substance of what has changed. What
exactly is the understanding that has been developed? How exactly
has the will been inspired? What exactly are the behaviors that
have emerged? Within this year-three evaluation, the participants

can claim the growth that has resulted from participating in the program and, by implication, the direction of their future growth. "Participants learn from each other"—this is clear from many of the session reports. The interpersonal context is crucial for developing the participants' capacities in the working knowledge and skills of leading the mission and ministry of Catholic Health Care. This aspect of the year-three evaluation will document the levels of support for the learning process from three different perspectives. Presently we obtain responses from the *cohort* colleagues (people who participated in the sessions together) and the *system* colleagues (participants from the same system). With the inception of several pilot projects, we are also obtaining responses from *non-program* colleagues who function within the same system as participants, but who have not attended MLC sessions.

There is a summary evaluation at the end of three years.

The summary evaluations at the end of the third year consist of some quantitative survey materials but are mostly qualitative in nature. We use a variety of formats to ask participants what they have learned and how they use it in their practice of health care. As the program adds more participants, this technique will produce an ever-growing body of reflection and articulation about how formation is practiced.

Assessing System-Level Formation Outcomes with Pilot Studies

There are two purposes of the pilot studies. First, we need to produce some objective measures of the results of formation, independent of the subjective view of the participants. Second, we need to develop information about the effects of the formation program within the systems managed by the participants. It is still too early to see broad systemic changes (the first wave of participants completed their course in 2008 and we are just now, in 2012, in a position to see a sufficient number of participants for analysis within some systems that have completed the course); but, it is possible to detect whether inroads are being made at the system level. To do this in a preliminary fashion, we propose combining the aggregated materials from the "personal" and "collegial" reflections with the qualitative overviews of the operation within each system. The salient issue for this portion of the evaluation is determining what the signs are that leadership within the system is following the direction set by the MLC formation program, what specific executive behaviors support this, and what the barriers are to further growth.

These three arenas of the year-three evaluation (personal, collegial, and systemic) generate "evidence by convergence" rather than in a prima facie manner. It is neither possible nor desirable at this early stage of the program to attempt a direct cause-and-effect evaluation. Nor is it wise to attempt to describe the outcomes of the program using "grades" or other such quantitative measures, because they are too narrow to capture the nature of growth in mature leaders and executives. Instead, the overall outcomes at this early stage are described in terms of the participants' expanded self-understanding about their role as leaders in Catholic Health Care and the aggregated evidence of what is happening within the systems that can be attributed to that expanded self-understanding.

MLC is currently participating in two "within-system" pilot projects using a technique of developing benchmark norms from existing MLC data and combining that with a review of existing formation data within the participating systems.

To the extent that all or most of the participants articulate personal growth using the language of the program, describe collegial discussions using that language, and refer to system activities congruent with the goals of the program, the systems are deemed to have started down a successful path of change in leadership formation. MLC is currently participating in two

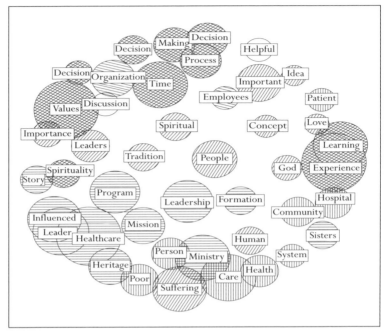

Figure 6.3 A word cloud

"within-system" pilot projects using this technique of developing benchmark norms from existing MLC data and combining it with a review of existing formation data within the participating systems. We are administering a baseline survey to all managers using a customized version of the Leadership Assessment Tool and will be monitoring leadership activities with the full consent of the managers and with the cooperation of the system executives. In addition, we are capturing written leadership articulations such as memos, decisions, and announcements. We will analyze these data using an "alignment index," which is produced with the Leadership Assessment Tool as the principle-dependent variable. We will review the final report with all the system stakeholders and produce a "state of leadership formation" document for use in their management planning activities.

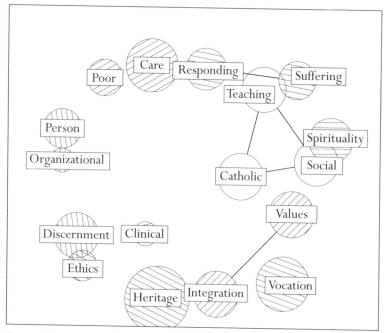

Figure 6.4 A redacted word cloud

The qualitative data are analyzed with word count frequency and sorting programs that incorporate both Linguistic Inquiry and Word Count (LIWC) programs and display programs from Provalis to produce dendrograms and word clouds that can be very analytically revealing. This process begins with counting the frequencies of terms (using LIWC) and then combines terms into conceptual descriptions using proximity analysis that measures the distance between words in a specific text. Greater or lesser proximity indicates conceptual and articulation patterns. For example, figure 6.3 is an initial word cloud for text that describes activities sorted into the area of the twelve foundational concerns. This process creates a description of both the "association between terms" (distance) and the "intensity of their use" (size of bubble). It depicts graphically the way participants articulate their experiences.

It can then be refined for clarity as seen in figure 6.4. These techniques will be used more and more as the base for analysis grows within participating systems. By combining qualitative and quantitative measures, we can keep the assessment practices current to match the formation experiences within the participating health care systems. As far as we know, MLC is currently the only formation program that has committed to ongoing assessment of such an extensive nature.

Design and Implementation of the Leadership Assessment Tool

The quantitative and qualitative data gathered over the past years have now been used to construct a Leadership Formation Assessment Tool that can be used with participating systems to evaluate executive leadership style against the benchmark of the twelve foundational concerns and the aggregated behaviors and attitudes of the seven hundred leaders that have completed the MLC program. This tool produces an "alignment index" that empirically reflects the congruence of the attitudes and practices of system leaders with the twelve MLC foundation concerns. This is an ongoing project that is modified as new data are produced by the MLC participants, but there is a core to the measurement index that can be used to construct valid time series analyses.

The Leadership Assessment Tool is based on the foundational concerns and the MLC Triangle, which are taught in the three-year program. It allows for the analysis of both quantitative and qualitative data generated by the program participants, and it can generate a variety of analytic reports to address the different concerns of the participating systems. This tool can generate a

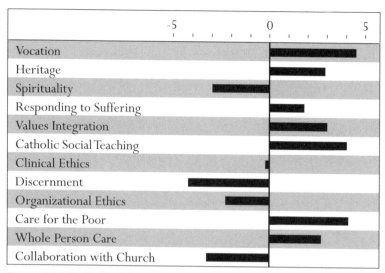

Figure 6.5 The leadership alignment index

report on the "personal growth in formation" that tracks an individual's development over the course of the program, and perhaps beyond. It can also generate a report on "formation within the system" that tracks the aggregated development of executives and managers with a specific system. Figure 6.5 is an example of an assessment of an individual's development in relation to the twelve foundational concerns. This person would be strong on "Vocation," "Catholic Social Teaching," and "Care for the Poor" and rather weak on "Spirituality," "Discernment," and "Whole Person Care."

Using a mix of qualitative and quantitative data allows for a broad evaluative perspective. The data flow from participants' articulations at the third-year summary session, in the online discussion forums on the website, and at the Action|Feedback sessions. Data are also captured from the session surveys and surveys during the program and with alumni. These data can produce individual profiles, system profiles, intersystem comparisons, and growth analyses. (See figure 6.6 for an example of the latter.) This would be a way to track development over several years.

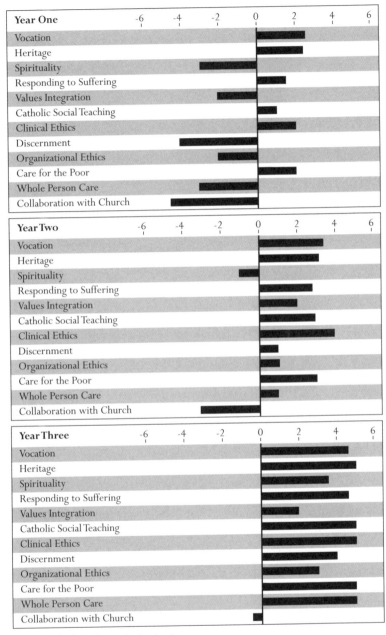

Figure 6.6 Growth analysis chart

The advantage of aggregating data for all participants is that we can establish norms for individuals and systems to use as benchmarks for the future. Here are typical questions that can be addressed: What types of leaders benefit most from the formation program? How has the growing cohort of MLC alumni affected specific systems? What system characteristics are related to successful formation? How have specific work groups benefited from MLC formation over time?

Conclusion

A formation program seeks to immerse individuals in a tradition for the purposes of continuing it. This general description has to be considerably qualified when it comes to the Catholic Health Care tradition, but it always entails a give and take between tradition and individual characteristics. On the one hand, the tradition has to be clearly and persuasively articulated. But on the other hand, the tradition has to be correlated with the consciousness and commitments of the individuals. Individuals and tradition mutually and continuously shape each other. Tradition can be presented coherently and abstractly, but when the individuals respond, a dialogue develops that has the potential to transform both. The overall purpose of the ongoing evaluation within MLC is to document this process with valid and reliable measurements.

When this general pattern is applied to formation programs for Catholic Health Care leaders, it suggests that the tradition can be reshaped by listening to leaders and that the leaders can be formed and reshaped by listening to the tradition. In a sense, this process mirrors the anthropologist's definition of culture as "webs of significance that we ourselves have spun."[3] MLC's leadership formation program is about leaders themselves "spinning webs of significance" that will nurture and support a new generation of Catholic Health Care leaders.

Notes

1. Everett M. Rogers, *Diffusion of Innovations* (New York: Free Press, 1983).

2. Clifford Geertz, *The Interpretation of Cultures: Selected Essays* (New York: Basic Books, 1973), 3–30.

3. Ibid., 5: "The concept of culture I espouse, and whose utility the essays below attempt to demonstrate, is essentially a semiotic one. Believing, with Max Weber, that man is an animal suspended in webs of significance he himself has spun, I take culture to be those webs, and the analysis of it to be therefore not an experimental science in search of law but an interpretive one in search of meaning."

CHAPTER 7

Formation, Technology, and Blended Learning

Diarmuid Rooney and Bill Fitzgerald

I was overcome by the dialogue we had online about this. I learned so much by sharing materials and looking back at our foundation [heritage] and our faith and beliefs and asking how these can help us continue our mission—as we engage the future. As one member said, although we need to remain faithful to our Catholic heritage, we need to also be able to creatively adapt this and engage the contemporary world put before us.

—MLC Participant

We live in the era of the social web, and interacting online has evolved into a mainstream practice. While the merits of this shift are debatable, it redefines how we understand interpersonal interactions. Formation is first and foremost a face-to-face process—relationship is its very *raison d'être.* The initial suggestion of engaging technology as part of formation was met with both resistance and skepticism. Four years later, after building and using a custom-designed website, this initial perspective has been reshaped due to MLC's experience supporting formation in an online space. As one MLC board member recently remarked, "It is impossible now to imagine MLC without this learning platform." In this chapter, we will discuss how technology connects the off-site and on-site worlds of leaders, and strengthens community and integration.

183

As a knowledge- and experiential-based educational institute, MLC manages a wealth of content and materials for the organization and its members. Before 2009, MLC staff managed materials largely through paper reproductions, shared drives on closed networks, and email attachments. To respond to the needs of its growing membership, MLC proposed developing an interactive website and an online content-management system. The initial directive from the MLC board was to build a modest, easy-to-use site and see what traction there would be—if any—from our members. Board members and other stakeholders cited abundant cautionary examples of dormant and decaying SharePoint-type sites.

From the outset, MLC participants have been actively involved alongside MLC staff in program design. Before building the initial version of the site, MLC staff engaged focus groups, surveyed selected stakeholders, and formed an intra- and intersystem committee to help with defining the goals of the website. From this input, we created some initial user stories, or definitions and understandings of who would use the site and what they wanted to do in the site. Cautiously, with minimum investment and a build-as-we-go approach, the first rendition of the MLC website was launched. Although a considerable amount of creative planning and input was required, it was still somewhat of a surprise that the initial website (1.0) proved to be such a success.[1] The site rapidly became an indispensable feature of our formation efforts. Despite this achievement it soon became apparent that we were building on a foundation that was never designed to hold this much weight. The continued positive feedback, combined with increased usage of the site, enabled MLC and its sponsoring

> We began to see the emerging potential for how face-to-face communal formation could be supported and served by online communities. This organic development was a major breakthrough in how MLC continues to envision the art of formation in a new era.

systems to legitimate an appropriate investment. We engaged an excellent website developer with a focus in online education, and continued to further track and refine the user experience.[2] We began to see the emerging potential for how face-to-face communal formation could be supported and served by online communities. This organic development was a major breakthrough in how MLC continues to envision the art of formation in a new era. The outcome has been the creation of a first-class, interactive, web-based learning platform that serves both as an expansive repository for the materials produced since 2005 and as the home of a number of learning applications specifically designed for use online. The updated website (2.0), built on the success and lessons learned from the initial version of the website, has quickly become an invaluable information resource, a place for reflective interaction, and a tool for tracking integration efforts among participants; a medium for continued formation for our alumni; and an exciting intersystem collaboration tool for deepening integration and knowledge in all our sponsoring systems.

The MLC Website—Our Path to the Future

The Ministry Leadership Center site (www.ministryleadership.net) includes extensive public pages serving the growing interest in the discipline of formation (see figure 7.1). These pages offer an excellent introduction to formation and include participants' comments and enthusiastic endorsements from the CEOs of each system (the majority of whom have completed or are in the program). Every MLC member has a password-protected individual user account. There are five different levels of access, including active participant, alumni, Formation Integration Team member, staff, and MLC board member. Each assigned role enables the user to interact with specifically designed work spaces that best meet the needs of that user group.

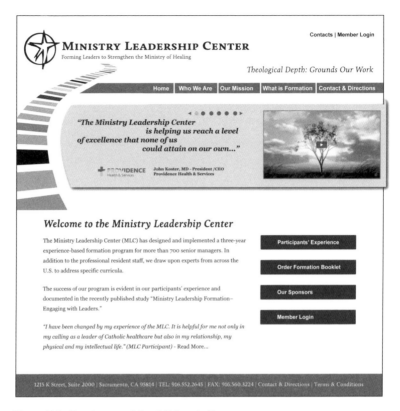

Figure 7.1 Front page of the MLC website

MLC Participant Experience

For the active participant, the site brings together multiple ways of learning interactively: curriculum for each of the twelve foundational concerns; an interactive social learning process named "Action|Feedback"; integration practice resources; and discussions, comments, and interactions between forum members. Each of these elements provides a means of studying, interacting with, and reflecting on ideas and practices relevant to formation; these elements focus on supporting participants as they implement these ideas and practices in their work. The individual elements all play a role in the formation process, but the most compelling

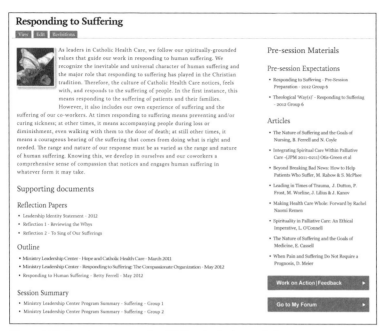

Responding to Suffering

View Edit Revisitions

As leaders in Catholic Health Care, we follow our spiritually-grounded values that guide our work in responding to human suffering. We recognize the inevitable and universal character of human suffering and the major role that responding to suffering has played in the Christian tradition. Therefore, the culture of Catholic Health Care notices, feels with, and responds to the suffering of people. In the first instance, this means responding to the suffering of patients and their families. However, it also includes our own experience of suffering and the suffering of our co-workers. At times responding to suffering means preventing and/or curing sickness; at other times, it means accompanying people during loss or diminishment, even walking with them to the door of death; at still other times, it means a courageous bearing of the suffering that comes from doing what is right and needed. The range and nature of our response must be as varied as the range and nature of human suffering. Knowing this, we develop in ourselves and our coworkers a comprehensive sense of compassion that notices and engages human suffering in whatever form it may take.

Supporting documents

Reflection Papers
• Leadership Identity Statement - 2012
• Reflection 1 - Reviewing the Whys
• Reflection 2 - To Sing of Our Sufferings

Outline
• Ministry Leadership Center - Hope and Catholic Health Care - March 2011
• Ministry Leadership Center - Responding to Suffering: The Compassionate Organization - May 2012
• Responding to Human Suffering - Betty Ferrell - May 2012

Session Summary
• Ministry Leadership Center Program Summary - Suffering - Group 1
• Ministry Leadership Center Program Summary - Suffering - Group 2

Pre-session Materials

Pre-session Expectations
• Responding to Suffering - Pre-Session Preparation - 2012 Group 6
• Theological 'Way(s)' - Responding to Suffering - 2012 Group 6

Articles
• The Nature of Suffering and the Goals of Nursing, B. Ferrell and N. Coyle
• Integrating Spiritual Care Within Palliative Care -(JPM 2011-0211) Otis-Green et al
• Beyond Breaking Bad News: How to Help Patients Who Suffer, M. Rabow & S. McPhee
• Leading in Times of Trauma, J. Dutton, P. Frost, M. Worline, J. Lilius & J. Kanov
• Making Health Care Whole: Forward by Rachel Naomi Remen
• Spirituality in Palliative Care: An Ethical Imperative, L. O'Connell
• The Nature of Suffering and the Goals of Medicine, E. Cassell
• When Pain and Suffering Do Not Require a Prognosis, D. Meier

Work on Action | Feedback ▶

Go to My Forum ▶

Figure 7.2 Session page on the MLC website for participants

gains are seen when the cumulative effects of both the face-to-face and virtual engagement are integrated both personally and organizationally by the participants over time. Within the site, participants can access all of the materials used in each of the twelve sessions covering the foundational concerns (see figure 7.2 for an example). These materials are always available, in their entirety, to all participants both during their time in the program and after their completion of the program. (After participants complete the program, they remain members of the site and can access the updated session materials as well as additional materials specifically designed for alumni.) Each session page includes a description of the session topic as well as links to all of the readings, exercises, and other documents relevant to that session. There are also pre-session materials that each participant is expected to complete before the session meeting, including specific readings and exercises that will be discussed at the session. In addition to the pre-session materials, there are supporting documents available for each session. All of the session presentations, summaries, and reflection papers remain available at all times, enabling ongoing integration efforts between sessions.

Tracking Ideas

As participants read through session materials, they can take notes and track ideas as they read by using the "notes" tab that appears on the side of the web page (see figure 7.3). When a participant takes a note, it is saved to their account, where they can retrieve it later. Participants can add a note by clicking on the "notes" tab; this slides open a panel on the left side of the screen where they can type notes about the page they are currently reading. Participants can add or edit notes at any time. Tracking ideas has always been an expectation of the program and it is now easier and more accessible than ever to do so.

Having access to materials and notes at all times means that participants can prepare for the face-to-face meetings when it works for them. Additionally, as part of the second iteration of the MLC site, all materials were made available and accessible via commonly used handheld devices, including smartphones and tablet computers. The emphasis on accessibility to the session materials—on devices including computers, smartphones, and iPads—means that people can access and read materials during short breaks when they have a small window of free time. Formation is a cumulative process where the emphasis is on personal consciousness change and the behaviors that will emerge from the change. This takes time and is one of the reasons why the program requires three years. A parallel concern to the formation process is how to meet the reality of an executive's hectic life regarding practical study, reflection, and sharing. By ensuring that the materials and resources are as accessible to as many participants in as

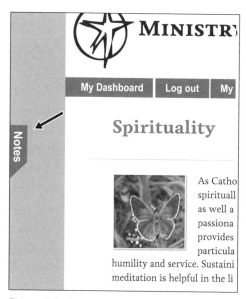

Figure 7.3 Online notes tool

many ways as is realistically possible, we remove barriers to access that often exist in less flexible learning systems. Additionally, if we look at accessibility to formation materials through the lens of supporting and increasing integration, having formation materials easily accessible via mobile devices that people are already using increases the likelihood that people will be thinking about and integrating these ideas within their normal workday and work routine. The ability to support the participant in this way led to a fundamental shift in using web media to dramatically increase integration efforts. The development and adaption of an existing verbal reporting tool—Action|Feedback—into an interactive social platform highlighted the potential for the creative marriage of technology and formation.

Action | Feedback—a Co-Creating Learning Tool

Action|Feedback is a learning activity designed to further support the formation process through building communities of practice both on-site (at the retreat center) and off-site (virtually). The Action|Feedback exercise enables participants to gain direct practical experience in the MLC core skills of "articulation and integration" as they engage these three simple questions between sessions: What did I do? What was the feedback? What did I learn? In other words, participants need to articulate the action they have taken, the feedback they have received, and what they have learned regarding the integration and application of what they have experienced in the off-site sessions (see figure 7.4). Action|Feedback has been an essential feature of the program from the very beginning (it was originally referred to as "off-site teaching"), and the online addition allows members to interact electronically in small forums between sessions. The online tool was designed and developed to complement the participant's experience; it was specifically created for leaders to be able to practice articulating how the knowledge conveyed at the sessions relates to their working situations and how this knowledge can be integrated into their personal and organizational life. We relied on the leaders themselves to inform us of what would best serve this goal, and it was through this essential partnership that the Action|Feedback process became a central feature of the formation process.

> The Action|Feedback exercise enables participants to gain direct practical experience in the MLC core skills of articulation and integration as they engage these three simple questions between sessions: What did I do? What was the feedback? What did I learn?

Action | Feedback—the Process

As discussed in previous chapters, each group has 120 people, which in turn has 3 cohorts of 40 people, and each cohort has

Action

What did you do?:

Please describe the situation. Please describe the process.

Presentation tips

Feedback

What was the feedback?:

Please describe the feedback you received. Please describe the process through which you received feedback.

Presentation tips

Lessons learned

What did you learn?:

Please describe what helped you learn during this process. Please describe some lessons learned as a result of this work that led to improvement.

Presentation tips

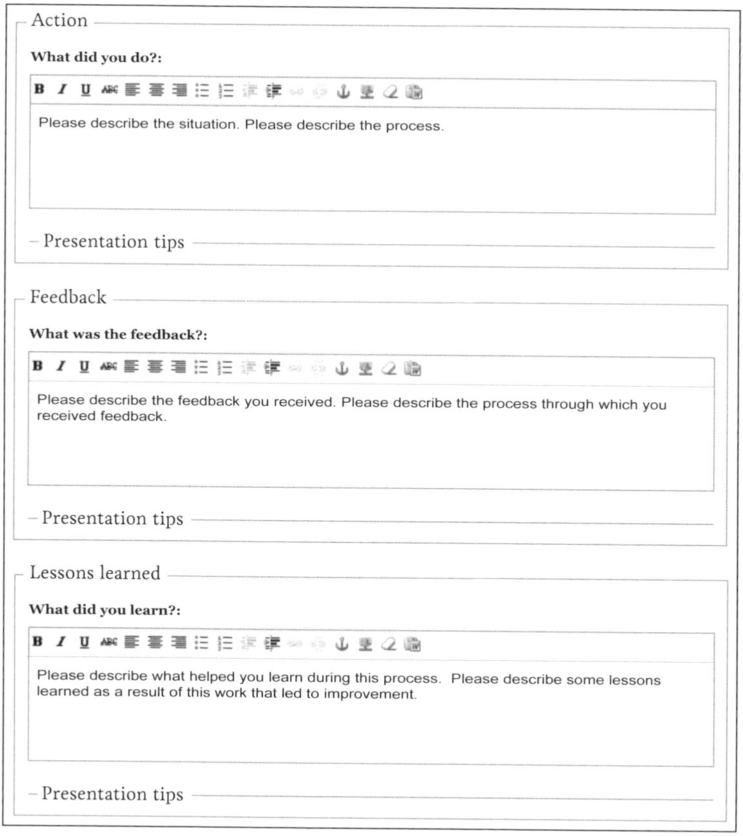

Figure 7.4 Action | Feedback page for participants

6 forums of 6 to 10 members. In the Action|Feedback process, each participant is assigned to a specific forum (see figure 7.5). The process always begins in person at the session; each forum has time together for sharing, discussing, and planning around what has been most exciting for each of them during the session. These conversations create opportunities for community building while participants prepare what they will do for their Action|Feedback in their organization. This is mediated at the session, in person, through concrete examples and a series of personal reflections. The personal reflections can begin in many ways: "Of all the

topics we talked about regarding session foundational concern, what interested me the most was . . ."—"When I think of sharing what interested me most about session foundational concern in an Action|Feedback session with a particular group or individual, I encounter the obstacle of . . ."—"When I think of sharing what interested me most about session foundational concern in an Action|Feedback with a particular group or individual, I envision the benefit of . . ." After participants have engaged in their personal reflections, they discuss next steps within their forum using these sentence: "Describe the Action|Feedback opportunity you are thinking about and the action you will take."—"When you are listening, imagine you are a participant in the process you are hearing about . . . and give concrete feedback." During the face-to-face sessions at the retreat center, participants work within their forums to prepare for integration opportunities in their work. Then, as participants return to their sites, the forums continue conversations and collaborations online, enabling peer learning through dialogue, sharing of integration practices, and growth of knowledge.

Online Formation Collaboration

Directly after each session, all forum members receive an email notification that prompts them to begin their individual Action|Feedback and gives them the submission deadline. This includes a link to their "dashboard" on the site, where they get a complete overview of all the most recent session materials (including any notes they may have taken electronically). (See figure 7.6.) We provide them with concrete Action|Feedback examples. They can also see all the previous submissions that they and other cohort members have created. For example, one participant wrote on the Vocation foundational concern for their Action|Feedback, "I was surprised to find how much I resonate with the idea that the work I do every day is my calling. I decided to introduce the

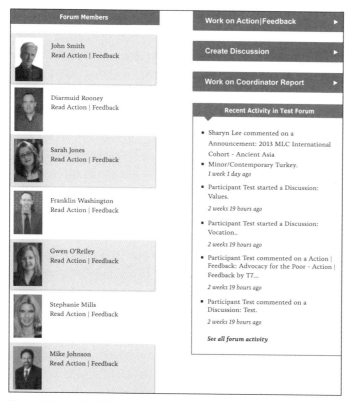

Figure 7.5 Action I Feedback forum members

topic and begin a discussion around vocational attitude/calling with my direct reports. As part of the performance appraisal [PA] process, I requested written input and discussion around this theme regarding things they are most proud to have accomplished, how goals were met and the establishment of new goals. I have now included a discussion about vocational attitude in the PA process."

Once they have submitted their most recent Action|Feedback, all of the other forum members receive an email notification and forum members can read and comment on the work of their peers. This allows for immediate feedback, interaction, and sharing of resources. The work and comments of members are shared privately within their forum, generating a level of trust and openness. (An MLC staff moderator is always included and available in all forums.)

After all participants within a forum have completed their Action | Feedback, the forum coordinator (a rotating position that is shared among all the forum members) prepares a summary of all the forum members' work that highlights the key learnings that occurred. For example, here is an excerpt from a forum coordinator report on the foundational concern Organizational Ethics: "We (as a Forum) realized that we have to get *all* the information regarding the situation. We need to hear both sides so an intelligent and fair decision can be made that is ethically sound and correct. It was also noted (by a forum member) that it is important that the right people with the right tools are involved in developing a solution. These types of decisions cannot be made in a vacuum and it takes a team of people working together to come up with a solution that is for the greater good. The process *must* be communicated properly for the decision to be fully understood and integrated in the organization." Once the forum coordinator prepares and posts an initial draft of the report, forum members are notified and can provide additional dialogue and feedback, usually resulting in edits and revisions. In this way, with the feedback provided by forum members, the draft version of the forum coordinator report is prepared. (This will ultimately be presented to the larger cohort.) This online community activity generates virtual dialogue around formation issues and creates a sense of ownership around the report that can lead to very novel and creative presentations to the larger cohort, which is part of the next aspect of the Action | Feedback process, shared learnings.

Action | Feedback Shared Learnings

At the following face-to-face session, the forums reconvene (at a designated time) to discuss their experiences and to finalize the forum coordinator's report. The forum coordinator facilitates the

Forum Navigation
Session Materials
Forum Discussions
Action | Feedback Examples
Action | Feedback Submissions
Forum Coordinator Report not ready
All Forum Coordinator Reports
Get Help

Upcoming A|F Dates
Forum coordinator: Jack Shea
Active session: Discernment
Start date: 2011-12-08
Coordinator edits: 2011-12-19
Completion date: 2011-12-16
Next meeting: 2012-04-10
Next Session Module:

Figure 7.6 Forum members dashboard

dialogue where each forum member gets a chance to speak about any additions to what they did and learned. There is a sentence stem to focus the forum: "This forum would like to tell the whole cohort about this particular learning which is important for our skills of articulation and integration." Each of the forum coordinators gives a short presentation on the learnings within their forum to the rest of the cohort. This gives each participant the opportunity to further practice the skill of articulation. For example one participant shared the following from their Action|Feedback on the foundational concern on Spirituality: "our ministry recently experienced a reduction in force that was difficult for everyone. In a meeting with my direct reports, I elected to spend an hour to decompress from the events of the last week and bring us all in touch with what sustains us during challenging times. I utilized the Defeating and Sustaining Spirit exercise to aid us in the discussion. We brainstormed those experiences that can either defeat our sense of spirit or sustain us. We talked in depth about what each of those experiences was and how they impacted our spirit so the group could appreciate each other's triggers. I realized in the course of the exercise that the discussion itself was sustaining and restoring my own spirit. The group was investing in each other to build each other up and positively face another day as leaders of the ministry." The participants have said that it is also very helpful for people to witness their peers engaging in this process. While it may seem obvious, cohort members are given explicit instructions to listen for relevant sections of the forum coordinator's reports. This pragmatic, focused listening helps participants glean specific details that they can subsequently integrate into their specific work situations. The presentations vary and often involve handouts of best practices for integration; on occasion, we have enjoyed original songs and videos!

After each report out, participants can ask questions and discuss points of interest. After the final report, there is also time for what we call "The Marketplace of Ideas." Members of the forums (and all the MLC staff) are invited to gravitate to the tables where they heard details that interested them; in smaller groups, they are able to pursue areas of interest in greater depth. This activity has an open-ended, almost fair-like atmosphere. People drag chairs around, stand around tables, and move from table to table, depending on what they want to hear or what appears interesting. It is a great community-building exercise where we often find people in similar roles (chief operating officers, chief nursing officers, and so on) gather to share integration practices around what they have heard. Over time, the best practices from these reports will become a searchable formation integration resource library for all MLC members.

Additional Benefits and Supportive Features

The immediate benefit of the online interactions is that people come into the face-to-face meetings familiar with—and prepared to discuss—their learning in the previous session.[3] Additionally, despite not having seen one another since the last face-to-face meeting, participants can feel a level of familiarity that—because of their the virtual communications—allows them to create trusting, supportive communities more quickly. In this way, the face-to-face and the online interactions become mutually supportive, and the combination allows participants to become more immersed in a supportive community of fellow participants experiencing the formation process. Additionally, all of the dialogue around Action|Feedback and forum coordinator reports remains online and—like the session materials—is always available to participants. Over time, this creates a body of knowledge and interactions that allows participants to track their growth and learning within the program. This all helps inform the annual leadership statements that each participant has to complete for the program, all of which, again, are available to them in their personal account on the MLC website.

It is worth noting that the site also provides different methods for various types of communication and reflection. Participants can start discussions with their forum members at any time. Unlike Action|Feedback, which is a structured opportunity showing how the ideas and practices from a specific formation topic were integrated into their personal and professional lives, and the forum coordinator's report, which is a summary highlighting the learning of forum members, discussions are rooted in the questions, comments, and thoughts of participants. Because participants can start discussions at any time, for any reason, they allow for open conversations about any subject. The addition of discussions—along with the ability to comment on Action|Feedback and forum coordinator's reports—aids in participants feeling a sense of ownership of and belonging within their forum. This, in turn, helps build the community bonds that get further reinforced and strengthened during the regular in-person meetings. It is well known that many sites have been brought live to serve as repositories for content, and these sites, predictably, remain completely static and underused. Since the MLC site provides participants with a range of ways to interact around the formation materials and to get feedback on any questions in close to real time, participants have many ways to communicate with one another around the questions that arise as part of formation. This shift transforms the way people use the site, from a simple source of content into a place where they can really connect, where relationship, the key to all formation, is nourished and deepened.

A Work in Progress

While the process for Action|Feedback continues to be an organic co-creation with many learnings along the way, it has become an integral part of our work. Participants spend up to three hours at each session unpacking and sharing the work they have done virtually in their forums, exchanging best practices (intra- and intersystem), and preparing practically for what they are going to focus on from the session for their personal and organizational integration efforts. The clear outcomes have been increased individual accountability; increased ability to find a voice, to articulate the foundational concerns of Catholic Health Care; and increased integration in both the system and local organizations. The rate of submissions of Action|Feedback work averages to around 92 percent across the groups (each has 120 people). Obviously we aim for 100 percent but we have been repeatedly informed (by web-blended learning consultants) that this participation rate is remarkable high, and that it suggests an excellent level of engagement and reflects the fact that the site is particularly user-friendly.

> The clear outcomes of the Action|Feedback process have been: increased individual accountability; increased ability to find a voice to articulate the foundational concerns of Catholic Health Care; increased integration in both the system and local organizations.

Learnings along the Path

One of the three MLC core values is relevance; we constantly depend on the insight and expertise of our members to keep our work relevant to the day-to-day experience and the needs of leadership. The initial version of the site brought together several elements that had been identified as critical in stakeholder interviews. These elements included a single, easily accessible place to access formation materials and a single place for forums to share Action|Feedback and forum coordinator reports. As participants began using the site, they expressed the desire to have more ways to interact within their forums, which led to opening up comments on Action|Feedback and forum coordinator reports. Creating a space for participants to provide feedback, and for that feedback to be implemented in the site, has contributed to high rates of participation within the site.

As the site has evolved, the types of interactions within the site have shifted. In the first version of the site, the use of the site and conversations within the site were largely focused on discussions of single units. Past sessions, while still available, were difficult to access, and linking work from past sessions to current sessions was problematic. In the second version of the site, the presentation of past work shifted to provide a balanced emphasis on the formation materials and the various points of conversation between people in forums. This shift—from reading and reacting to content, to reading and sharing a response to that content within the forum—marked a major shift in the types of interactions within the site.

As the complexity and frequency of online interaction increased, the presence of a skilled "former and community moderator" played an increasingly crucial role in the evolution of these online interactions between participants. During in-person sessions, as participants undertake the work required to experience and engage the formation process, they receive the support, structure, and guidance provided by the MLC staff. The same mechanisms are required for the online formation process. A skilled formation professional is essential for supporting and moderating the online dialogues and for reviewing the submissions and simply for being present for the MLC members. Life in all its complexity, joys, and sorrows is constantly unfolding for people participating in the program. This lived reality combined with the very subject matter of formation necessitates a skilled, supportive, and mature ear combined with an understanding of the world of the health care executive. Practically the participants (and especially the forum coordinators) need additional support as they navigate not only the new technology but also the new language that they are learning. This "former" has multiple roles, especially in a small organization, ranging from technological development to administrative support; ultimately, this person helps provide a measure of stability and a sense that help is never more than an email or an online discussion away.

> As the complexity and frequency of online interaction increased, the presence of a skilled "former and community moderator" played an increasingly crucial role in the evolution of these online interactions between participants.

Using Technology to Extend Integration

The MLC website and the face-to-face meetings for all our MLC members are now integrated components of a coherent process, one that is much bigger than the initial three-year program. We have primarily focused here on how we use technology to support the active participants. However, four other stakeholder groups within MLC also use the website to support their ongoing integration work—alumni, the Formation Integration Team, MLC staff, and the MLC board. All of these groups have specific work spaces designed to support their interests. After a participant has completed the three-year program, they transition to being alumni. The alumni have access to all the new active participant materials and many other valuable formation resources (see figure 7.7).

200

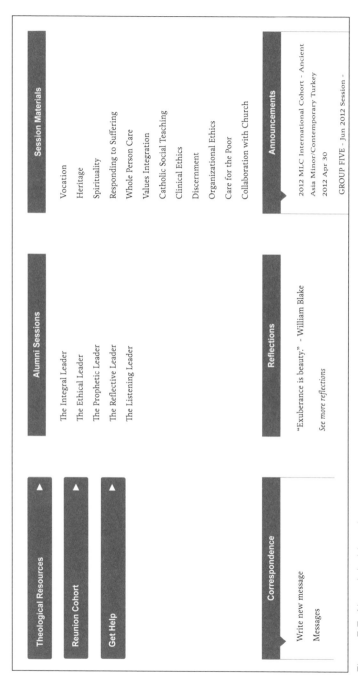

Figure 7.7 Alumni dashboard

More on the interactive exercise

Thu, 2012-07-19 09:19

Hi all,

Jack Shea

Ellen, could you tell us a little more about the interactive exercise and the feedback. Thanks.

delete   edit   reply

Values integration

Thu, 2012-07-19 10:22

Hi Jack:

Ellen Garcia

The Exercise was very simple and modeled after our daily practice. At each one of my employee forums, I asked team members to break into small groups of six-eight individuals. I mentioned that I'd been reflecting on the value of excellence on a daily basis as part of my values integration work inspired by ministry formation. I asked team members to reflect back on the past week and share a time when they onserved the value of excellence in action. Folks then reported back to the larger group. At the close, I asked everyone to notice the amount of energy this discussion created and invited them to take a moment each day to acknowledge excellence in other team members and in themselves.

This exercise touched about 200 employees -- from various disciplines ranging from caregivers, housekeeping, drivers, parmacisis, nurses, social workers, therapists, physicians and others. I received very positive feedback from those who participated.

Thanks again for leading us on our journey to "turn the wheel" daily.

Aloha, Ellen

delete   edit   reply

Thanks, Ellen

Thu, 2012-07-19 11:58

There is something in us, people, that wants to do our best, have it contribute, and have it acknowedged.

Jack Shea

delete   edit   reply

Figure 7.8

An example of a discussion between a staff member and a participant

In addition to continued access to the core formation session material, we developed interactive video tutorials specifically designed around the needs of those who completed the three-year program. Each tutorial consists of four five-minute dialogues between members of the MLC team and a leading figure in a particular area of concern for Catholic Health Care. Each five-minute segment can be viewed individually or in sequence, and each section is followed by a formation question. We developed the tutorials in response to requests for more support in ongoing formation and MLC's learning that the further you get from the formation experience itself the more diluted the process becomes. The alumni tutorials have been designed for easy use with executive teams or other groups in the organization. Examples topics include "The Integral Leader," "The Ethical Leader," "The Prophetic Leader," and "The Reflective Leader." To support ongoing formation and integration work within systems, MLC has also developed a section for theological resources. In this section of the website, we offer materials on three areas of interest:

- Theological "Why(s)": The theological importance of the twelve foundational concerns of Catholic Health Care that we cover in the formation process.

- Theological Perspectives: Audio podcasts on the theological grounding of key topics of importance to leaders of the ministry. Three podcasts are now available: "Mission Statements," "Values," and "Diversity." Several more are in development.

- Reflections: Resources developing personal and organizational reflection.

All of these applications on the website complement and support the face-to-face, biannual alumni reunion cohorts.

The website also provides an extensive platform for the MLC staff to engage with MLC members at multiple levels. All the members' dashboards include recent staff announcements and our

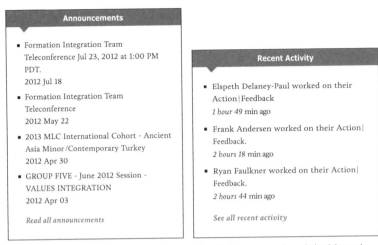

Announcements

- Formation Integration Team
  Teleconference Jul 23, 2012 at 1:00 PM
  PDT.
  2012 Jul 18
- Formation Integration Team
  Teleconference
  2012 May 22
- 2013 MLC International Cohort - Ancient
  Asia Minor / Contemporary Turkey
  2012 Apr 30
- GROUP FIVE - June 2012 Session -
  VALUES INTEGRATION
  2012 Apr 03

Read all announcements

Recent Activity

- Elspeth Delaney-Paul worked on their
  Action | Feedback
  1 hour 49 min ago
- Frank Andersen worked on their Action |
  Feedback.
  2 hours 18 min ago
- Ryan Faulkner worked on their Action |
  Feedback.
  2 hours 44 min ago

See all recent activity

Figure 7.9 Announcements and recent activity on members' dashboard

quarterly MLC Executive Director's eNewsletter. With the active participants, we are constantly uploading new formation materials for review and extending hyperlinked bibliographies. With the alumni, we continue to develop rich and relevant content for the interactive video tutorials and podcasts. We also are able to interact with members through private correspondence (there is an email facility on the site), through comments on their Action|Feedback, and by creating general discussions. (See figure 7.8 for an example.) Staff receive notification whenever there is activity in the site and can see all the recent activity. (See figure 7.9.)

As the programs offered within MLC continue to evolve, the platform will continue to grow and evolve to support the people doing the work. In building the website, we have been careful to balance current needs against the need for future growth and expansion. In the next year, MLC will develop additional resource The interactions supported by the website will continue to be informed by the work performed by people within the site. This ongoing co-evolution will help ensure that the skills of articulation and integration have a real and lasting impact.

Notes

1. Using Qualtrics, we did numerous surveys, completed a usability study, and listened carefully to all the input and advice from our users, which included comments that the site needed to be "even easier to navigate," that it needed to have "tighter technology across platforms to guarantee the quality of the users experience," and that it needed to have the "most professional user experience possible" (where all is seamless, where the website works with all browsers, and where the website is re-skinned to have a better, more slick appearance). Perhaps the most important feedback was from the person who said, "If I have a bad experience once, I am unlikely to use the medium again."

In addition, there were numerous suggestions for how to advance the site and what tools would enable an even better user experience. The technology at that time had been developed by a small, local boutique technology development studio (Grip Media), which continues to be intimately involved with the creative elements and tech support. While they had done an excellent job, they themselves pointed out to us that we (MLC) had grown beyond their capacity. Our needs were such that we needed to hire or contract a larger vendor for our growing technology expansion and needs; to develop interactive technologies that extend the technology into the mobile space for educational initiatives; to raise the interactive online tools to the highest level possible with current and emerging technologies; to develop the site for iPad and Tablet use, specifically for educational purposes; and overall to make navigation easier, the presentation of content better, and the use of screen real estate and consistent branding better.

2. Bill Fitzgerald, the executive director of Funny Monkey (www.funnymonkey.com), was our first consultant for the website, in collaboration with Jerry Chrisman and Grip Media. He was the author of *Drupal in Education*, which directly addressed two crucial needs for MLC, a Content Management System (CMS) and a blended formation and learning platform. Drupal is used by some of the biggest sites on the web, like The Economist, Examiner.com, and The White House. Those working at Funny Monkey are recognized national Drupal experts with portfolio examples including Teaching Tolerance (www.tolerance.org), Edutopia (www.edutopia), and the acclaimed National Writing Project website Digitails (www.digitalis.nwp.org). In 2010, they were recipients of major grant funding from the Knight Foundation to build Voice Box, an application that enables users (primarily communities and educational institutes) to share, publish, and interact across multiple media. Fitzgerald subsequently was invited and agreed to serve as the Senior Fellow for Communities of Practices at the Ministry Leadership Center. He provides guidance on how to develop a community that bridges online interactions and face-to-face meetings specific to the formation process. Additionally, he helps with the strategic planning required to expand existing MLC programs to a broader audience within the six sponsoring systems.

3. The following is a concise list of the website technological features and development:

- cloud-based note taking: an internal note-taking application for individuals; people can take notes on session materials as they prepare for in-person meetings and as part of their Action|Feedback;

- Scribd: a Web 2.0 document-sharing application that allows immediate access to documents of various formats, creating easier access to information within the site;

- Apache Solr search: a robust internal site search that allows site members to find more relevant information with less work;

- modular design: each component of the site is designed to allow for customization, depending on user needs;

- high capacity: the ability to handle thousands of independent users from multiple systems;

- responsive design: the content on the website "responds" to the screen size of the device upon which it is being viewed, which means that people can browse content on any device—from a smartphone to a tablet to a traditional computer—with an internet connection;

- better collaboration: the entire website design has been updated to foster increased collaboration and communication between formation participants;

- improved page-load times: the site design and graphics have been optimized for performance improvements; and

- streamlined design: clean, lightweight graphic design highlights the site content and supports interactions around that content.

CHAPTER 8

Facilitation/Resource in Leadership Formation

Mary Anne Sladich-Lantz

In the Ministry Leadership Formation Program, the group process begins by recognizing the established expertise of the participants in the diverse fields that comprise contemporary health care.[1] We address the participants in a way that acknowledges the rich professional education and years of experience they bring to the formation conversation. Our intention is to infuse what they already know and the work they do every day with the essential components of the twelve foundational concerns. To fulfill this intention, the formation must not become a course of study or set of knowledge; it must be an experience that can be fully integrated into the work of leaders in Catholic Health Care.

The process of facilitation assists the participants in their ability to articulate with grace and confidence the key components of each formation session. While presenting content that is grounded in the Catholic tradition and is consistent with current health care trends is important, learning only happens when the participants are able to reflect personally and talk together about the tradition's relevance to their lived experience. The role of the facilitation process is to connect the dots between what happens at the retreat center and the work that is part of the day-to-day life of these health care leaders. Though elementary in some ways, these connections need to be explicitly named. We want to help leaders find their own words to articulate their experience through inter-actions with one another in small and large group conversations in an environment that allows them to feel comfortable speaking about something when they may not feel completely qualified or confident in that discussion.

In this chapter, I will describe ten aspects of facilitation/resource we have learned or have found helpful as we guide and direct the formation process. They are listening over time, engaging the one speaking with the group, knowing the topic, creating a safe environment, affirming the speaker, inviting introverts, varying the process, calling an audible, recognizing uniqueness, and noting development. Many more techniques of facilitation/resource could be mentioned, but these ten are consistently used to guide the process.

Listening over Time

While each of the twelve sessions has a particular focus and can stand on its own in many respects, each is part of a whole. As the program progresses, participants are able to make connections from one session to another and often discuss what in the current session resonates with material from previous sessions. For example, during the session on Values Integration, participants often remember conversations from the session on Vocation/Call. As facilitators of this formation process, we should engage

> We assist the participants in determining where there is resonance, where they might feel some resistance, and where they might have questions or need further clarification.

with the participants to remember previous conversations in the large group and reference them. This engagement helps string the beads of the program together and create a sense of the whole. In addition, it reminds the participants that others hear their reflecting and sharing and that their contribution to the formation conversation is valuable.

Engaging the One Speaking with the Group

Facilitation of the formation process can be likened to an observed conversation between two people. When we enter into a large group discussion asking for comments from the participants, we never know where the conversation will take us. Once someone offers a thought or asks a question, the facilitator focuses directly on that person to listen for content and clarity. The large group discussion should allow each of the participants to practice articulating the subject matter and should help them deepen their overall learning. But in this interaction between the facilitator and the participant, the overall discussion must also be guided so that the whole group benefits. As one person shares thoughts or asks questions, the entire group should be led to a deeper place or to greater understanding. The facilitation process of moving from one person to the large group is like a dance with each movement leading to the next. The more graceful the interchange is, the greater the impact of the discussion will be.

Knowing the Topic

The facilitator needs to have a command of the subject matter to effectively lead the group to deeper understanding. As facilitators, we have an idea of where we want the conversation to go and what learnings we hope the participants will gain from the session. To facilitate at MLC, it is necessary to be well versed in the content of each session, to have a working knowledge of the Catholic tradition, and to be familiar with the current issues facing health care leaders. With this knowledge, the facilitator can reference this material and help the participants find how the session content is relevant to their particular experience. We assist the participants in determining where there is resonance, where they might feel some resistance, and where they might have questions or need further clarification.

Creating a Safe Environment

While we are not explicit in stating ground rules for the sessions, we do make the distinction between what is "personal private" and "personal public" in the first session, as we talk about the intended nature of our conversations together during the program. This distinction acknowledges that there are some things that are personal which may be inappropriate to share in a public setting and that there are other things that are certainly personal but are very appropriately shared in a public setting. Sharing personal experience, thoughts, and reflections about a given topic is essential to the overall purpose of the program, but participants are never asked to bare their soul to the group or to do anything that would make them feel uncomfortable. The nature of our learning environment is one of mutual respect, which allows the participants to explore their own responses to the subject matter presented. When the participants are confident that they will not be ridiculed or picked apart for what they ask or what they share, they are freer to engage in conversation. This type of personal safety is essential to the learning process. Facilitators set the tone by engaging with the participants in a way that allows them to stay open as they talk rather than shutting down for fear of saying something that does not make sense.

> The nature of our learning environment is one of mutual respect, which allows the participants to explore their own responses to the subject matter presented.

This "safe harbor" atmosphere allows the participants to experiment with the language of formation, which is not their first language.[2] They are quite competent and confident in talking strategy or finance or operations or the challenges of leading health care in these turbulent times. They have devoted a fair amount of time and resources to preparing themselves to be strong business leaders. However, once they enter the current world of Catholic

Health Care, they are asked to perform their professional role in a distinctive way. While many of our participants have a commitment to the mission of their particular organization, which some may even feel quite passionate about it, their ability to actually put that commitment or passion into words is not as developed. In our conversations with them, whether one-on-one during a break, while we roam from table to table during small group discussions, or when we talk together in the large group, we serve as guides in helping the participants find the right words to describe what they are coming to know as their own. The fruits of this guidance often become evident by the third year of the program. In the large group discussion during the session on Values Integration, which takes place in the final year of the program, we can point out to the participants how far they have come in their ability to articulate the principles of the foundational concerns covered to date. For two years, they are steeped in the language of the Catholic Health Care ethos and, without their conscious awareness, they begin to speak confidently about Catholic social teaching as it relates to the stated mission and core values of their organizations. Our providing an environment where the participants can try out this new language allows them to establish a command of the subject matter and a fluency in speaking about it.

Affirming the Speaker

Because all of our participants are leaders, one might assume that they are used to speaking in front of others and are self-assured. This is not always the case. Because of the subject, participants can feel a certain vulnerability when talking in the large group. As someone gets up the courage to speak, the attention of the facilitator naturally goes to that person with the intention of being completely engaged and supportive. While listening to the nature of the comment to determine the content and its relevancy to the topic at hand, it is necessary to give the person speaking some affirmation of their contribution. This affirmation takes the form of maintaining eye contact with the speaker, nodding to encourage them to continue, and offering a comment or two when they finish to let them and the group know that their contribution is valuable. Listening for feelings or personal opinions, in addition to content, also brings clarity to the discussion. Is there hesitance in the speaking? Does the speaker get emotional while making comments? Does the speaker seem uninterested or disengaged? Picking up on these nuances and using them to help unpack the conversation affirms the speaker in a subtle way. If the participants know that whatever they bring to the conversation is fine, they are more apt to connect at a deeper level with the subject.

> While listening to the nature of the comment to determine the content and its relevancy to the topic at hand, it is necessary to give the person speaking some affirmation for their contribution.

Sometimes the one speaking in the large group says something or presents a scenario that may be off base or may not be completely accurate. This situation requires extra effort to ensure that the facilitator, while using the comments as a teaching opportunity for the whole group, helps maintain the self-esteem of the speaker. For example, in the early years of the program, before the more formal Action|Feedback process began, participants were asked how they might bring the content of the session back to their teams. On one occasion, a bright, sincere, young CFO indicated that he intended to bring his team together for an all-day retreat that he would lead. We, of course, want all of the participants to share their formation experience and the knowledge they gain when they return to the workplace, and on the surface, this seemed like a noble thing to do. But because of our knowledge as facilitators, we knew that without some further conversations about how the retreat day would come to be, it was doomed to fail. In working through the difficulties of his plan with him in the presence of the rest of the group, the entire group began to learn from this CFO's enthusiasm how to share what they were learning with their team. We began the conversation by saying, "Would you be willing to explore your idea with the whole group?" When he said he would, we began asking him a series of questions: "Where do you plan to hold this retreat?" "How many people will be in attendance?" "How will you organize the day?" "What in particular do you think will have relevance for your team?" "Have you done something like this with your team before?" As we examined the details of having a day-long retreat, the CFO and the entire group gained clarity and insight about how to effectively put on such an event. By the time we finished the conversation, we concluded together that perhaps two to four hours would be better than a full day and we were able to help the CFO think through how to present his new found passion for the topic at hand to his team who may not have any familiarity with it. At no time during this interchange did the CFO feel like what he had considered was a really dumb idea. We affirmed his idea while showing a better way to act on his excitement.

Inviting Introverts

To use a common saying, extroverts talk to think while introverts think to talk. Extroverts are usually ready to speak immediately, needing little time to think about what they want to say. Introverts need some time to gather their thoughts before they can present them in conversation. If in a group, following a presentation, the facilitator immediately engages the group in conversation, then very likely the group will only hear from the extroverts. In facilitation at MLC, we acknowledge that introverts need time to think before speaking and we give the group a few minutes of silence to gather their thoughts and write down their

> Extroverts talk to think while introverts think to talk.

questions. Only then do we open the conversation to the whole group. This simple pause creates greater group participation.

Varying the Process

Our participants tell us in informal discussions that one of the most significant and valuable parts of the formation program is the sense of community they build with one another. While this undoubtedly happens on breaks, during meals, and at the social events, the development of community is facilitated by the meaningful sharing of personal experience in response to the foundational concern presented. To build community and hasten meaningful sharing, we develop exercises that help the participants think through the presenter's discussion and that assist them in working with the material personally and practically. In this development, we have found that when there is more variation in the exercises, the group is more engaged and the conversation is more meaningful. Our default mode is to provide questions for discussion or sentence stems for completion to be talked about at tables of five to eight participants and then to discuss those table conversations in the large group. This exercise allows participants to glean shared wisdom and to determine convergences. But there are many other useful exercises, some of which may be better suited for a particular subject. For example, in the session on Responding to Suffering, we invite the participants to share their experience of suffering in dyads because the sharing is much more intimate. In this situation, we do not ask them to share the conversation in the large group, but we do ask them to share their experience of having that kind of conversation. During the session on Spirituality, we also use the dyad model; but in this session, we invite them to take a walk outside to talk about practices they engage in that help keep them centered or grounded. Sometimes, we forgo the small group discussion in favor of having the conversation solely in the large group. Other times, we invite the participants to discuss at tables without bringing them back for a large group conversation. In the session on Vocation, we read together a series of five stories or experiences from the current literature to help the participants get a greater sense of what it means to enhance an attitude of call at work.[3] After the reading, each table is assigned one of the stories to discuss and a large group conversation follows the small group conversations. In the session on Values Integration, participants are asked in their work before the session to select from a list of topics in their assigned reading an area they would like to discuss.[4] At the session, they are divided according to interest group to discuss the topic in depth and to gener- ate insights and strategies that are then reported back to the whole group. The facilitation process moves from information received from a presentation, a video clip, or assigned work, to personal reflection on that information, to talking about it with others. Often we have a plan for how we will engage the group with the materials presented, but sometimes as we work with the group, we decide in the moment the best way to work with the material.

> In this development, we have found that when there is more variation in the exercises, the group is more engaged and the conversation is more meaningful.

Calling an Audible

A term from football, an "audible" is when the quarterback changes the play immediately before it takes place, usually in response to a sense that the play originally called will not be suitable, chang- ing the play at the line of scrimmage after reading the defense. In a similar way, we make it a practice to read the group and to determine in the moment the best way to work with the pre- sented material. We always come prepared with a detailed plan, but if the plan is not in sync with the group, those in the group will not be able to engage in a meaningful way. The day's agenda, the schedule, and the exercises we prepare serve as a guide not a harness. Our ability to be flexible and to respond to the needs of the group as we experience it ensures that the intended outcome of the session is met.

Recognizing Uniqueness

Each formation group is made up of three cohorts. As a result, every session is presented three times, usually over two weeks. While each cohort is at the same place in the three-year program and is made up of people from similar professional backgrounds and roles, the dynamics of each group are always distinct. The content of the three sessions is the same and we address each cohort with a similar intention in each session, but no two sessions end up being alike. Each cohort develops its own personality, and we work to interact with the group personality in ways that work best for them. Some groups seem to engage in an animated way at tables, so much so that we have a hard time ending the conversation; but when we invite conversation in the large group for these same groups, not much happens. For other cohorts, the opposite occurs. Assessing the group's personality and needs and adjusting the flow of the process accordingly adds to the overall success of the session.

Noting Development

Each session is crafted with the participants in mind. Health care leaders are used to a fast-paced, intense environment with any number of issues coming at them at any given time. They are used to multitasking (for better or worse) and are called on to perform the tasks of their job with efficiency and precision while making sure that the people who report to them feel valued and tended to. There is little time for pause, let alone to be reflective about the happenings of the day. Once our participants become accustomed to the flow of each session, they often comment on how grateful they are for this opportunity. For the most part, they come with an openness to engage with the content of each particular session. As the program has developed, we have been committed to keeping the didactic presentation to no more than thirty minutes, which is followed by an opportunity for participants to think individually and explore together where there is resonance for them and where there may be a rub or a conflict, as well as to ask questions. For some participants the opportunity to participate in the formation experience is seen as a tremendous privilege from the beginning, and what they have known to be true and have experienced in their personal and professional lives is affirmed by the content and the process of formation. As these participants move through the three-year process, they find themselves renewed in their commitment to serve their organization's mission and are more grounded in who they are and what they have to contribute. For others, it might take time to understand the meaning and the impact of the formation experience in their lives. Some have commented that they begin to get it somewhere around the fifth or sixth session. Almost every participant reports that there is a sense of sadness or loss as the program comes to an end because they have grown to appreciate the discipline of going off-site every quarter to learn and to reflect with their cohort. While three years seems like a very long commitment at the beginning of the program, it does not seem long enough at the end. The ongoing challenge we face is how to keep the formation conversation alive once the formal program is completed.

Conclusion

Certainly, there are skills to be learned for the process of facilitation, but mostly it is about the artful practice of engaging fully with the group of leaders sitting in front of us. It is an artful practice—a dance—of listening and responding and leading and guiding and learning together. But skilled facilitators do not just happen. Not all gifted presenters are able to effectively engage the group in discussing the information shared. Not everyone possesses the personal characteristics necessary for guiding a group in deepening the learning experience and engaging in dialogue. Our overall formation effort depends a great deal on the quality of the facilitation that takes place during each of the twelve sessions. For organizations interested in developing a formation program similar to ours, it would be important to make sure that someone with the gift and skills of facilitation is on the team.

The process of facilitation might be likened to that of a midwife. We believe that there is incredible new life continuing to be birthed in our midst as the work of Catholic Health Care continues to evolve in the absence of the founding communities of sisters and brothers.

The work of formation happens with the forty or so leaders gathered to engage in the socialization process of Catholic Health Care with one (or more) facilitators in front of them directing their work and guiding the conversation. The process of facilitation might be likened to that of a midwife. We believe that there is incredible new life continuing to be birthed in our midst as the work of Catholic Health Care continues to evolve in the absence of the founding communities of sisters and brothers. When we see the eyes of our participants shine with new insight and with a deep conviction that their work is making a contribution greater than they ever thought possible, there is no greater joy.

Notes

1. The Ministry Leadership Center defines formation as "a process of socialization into the community and tradition of Catholic health care for the purpose of building up the community and carrying on the tradition. It begins by recognizing the established expertise of the participants in the diverse fields that comprise contemporary health care. These health care professionals are then invited into a formation experience that centers on the twelve foundational concerns that inform the distinctive identity and mission of Catholic health care."

2. For further discussion on the topic of leaders finding their own mission "voice," see John O. Mudd, "From CEO to Mission Leader," *Health Progress*, September-October 2005, 25–27. In this article, the author acknowledges that current Catholic Health Care leaders are already proficient as business people but says that they must learn to be mission-literate as well. Not only do these leaders need to learn this second language but they must become eloquent in it as well.

3. The five stories used for group discussion in the first session on Vocation all come from current writing on finding meaning and purpose or joy in everyday life and at work. Each one presents a different perspective on how attitude affects one's overall experience. The group is led to unpack the stories so that they can gain greater insight into how they might grow in their own sense of call and how they might create an atmosphere in their own workplace that promotes an attitude of call.

4. For the session on Values Integration, the participants are given two articles to read as preparation. One comes from Keshavan Nair, *A Higher Standard of Leadership: Lessons from the Life of Gandhi* (San Francisco: Berrett-Koehler, 1997); the other is Jim Collins, "Aligning Values and Actions," *Forum*, June 2002. We divide the two articles into six areas of interest.

CHAPTER 9

System Cooperation and Collaboration in Leadership Formation

Elizabeth McCabe

This chapter discusses Intersystem Cooperation and Collaboration, the ways in which the Ministry Leadership Center (MLC) works with member systems to ensure deep integration of the formation experience within, across, and among systems. We will explore this cooperation and collaboration by examining the genesis of MLC as a fruit of collaboration, the history and evolution of MLC intersystem initiatives, the importance of key strategic partners, and the current approaches to intrasystem and intersystem integration, with a brief exploration of lessons learned and emerging concerns related to ongoing cooperation and collaboration.

Genesis of the MLC Collaboration

MLC came to life out of a coalition drawn from five Catholic health systems seeking a collective strategy to support strengthening and safeguarding their respective ministry's fidelity to the meta-story of Catholic Health Care. This coalition recognized its vital role and sought an intentional way, through the leadership of their respective ministries, to actively participate in a changing and pluralistic community committed to carrying forward a distinct revelation about a particular way to be in the world. The visionary inception of MLC grew out of an acknowledgment by the member systems that their collective mission integration efforts could most effectively take root and bear fruit if approached in a way that recognized both the commonality of the ministry across many systems and the distinct cultural aspects of each system. Not only is the genesis story of MLC reflective of the value and importance of collaborative innovation, but it also underscores an MLC hallmark grounded in a commitment to being attentive to our role and relationship to each member system. MLC is designed to ensure that the formation experience is in service to the transformative cultural intention of each system. The MLC formation experience is rooted in a dynamic interplay between the MLC program and responsiveness to system realities. (See figure 9.1.) Therefore, MLC relies on an essential partnership with each system. Our system integration work has historically supported, and is currently poised to support, each member system's initiative in order to leverage their leaders' formation experience for the broader organization, as well as to encourage collaborative work among the systems.

MLC is designed to ensure that the formation experience is in service to the transformative cultural intention of each system.

Intent and Purpose of System Integration Focus

The original intent and purpose of the MLC system integration focus included (a) consulting the sponsor systems so that they would provide support specific to MLC participants and alumni, (b) coordinating resources to support the enhancement and development of intrasystem formation initiatives, and (c) facilitating intersystem collegiality and collaboration. The value of focused attention on intra- and intersystem integration has always been identified as essential to meeting the intent of MLC, namely, to "form leaders to sustain and deepen the ministry of healing." We came to a formation

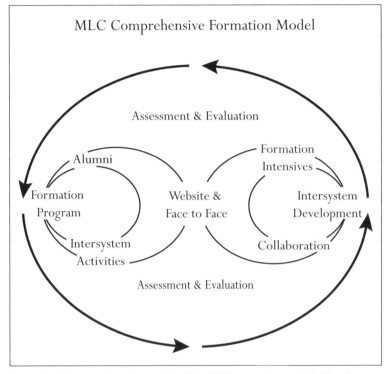

Figure 9.1 Comprehensive model of the MLC experience, including the programs and the intersystem dimensions

theory out of a formation practice; similarly, the refinement of a system integration theory is emerging from an increasing awareness of the importance of identifying intrasystem integration models of best practice and fostering intersystem collaboration. We began with a keen interest in the cultural distinctiveness of each system, the lived experience of formation within the system, and the varied intrasystem history and practices of formation.

System Integration Relies on Strategic Partners

Our essential partnership in system integration with member systems has been primarily with and through executive system leaders with accountability for mission integration and formation initiatives within member systems. These partners are able to contribute practically to the continued development of our endeavor to be attentive to integration, particularly during this unprecedented time within each member system, as well as in Catholic Health Care as a whole. These system-leader partners are actively leading and shaping system-specific responses to change and bring insight to collaborative dialogue on model strategies specific to Catholic Health Care beyond the specifics of their own systems. Because of their system accountability to strategic planning and the operationalization of mission, vision, and core values, they recognize the value of the MLC intersystem model of sustained formation, as well as the critical value and need to support the ongoing formation experience through thoughtful and strategic intra- and intersystem integration. Success in driving intrasystem initiatives that promote a symmetry between internal initiatives and MLC as well as in leveraging collective knowledge and practice among systems drives the need to select strategic partners of this caliber, who respond daily to practical concerns and realities and who join together to begin the dialogue about the system integration of formation.

System Diversity of Culture and Formation Practice

Each partner system within MLC has a distinct culture and is situated in a distinct reality related to intrasystem formation. For example, St. Joseph Health has a well-established formal formation program, Mission and Mentoring, which was in place before the inception of MLC and in fact served as a resource for identifying the twelve foundational concerns. Its fifteen-year experience of managing and integrating system-wide formation through this program provided a perspective and a platform on which they could build as the system engaged MLC. Other member systems with less system-wide formation in place are building programs with the advantage of St. Joseph Health's experience. While every system had formation elements inherent in new-employee orientation and practices such as meeting reflections, each was at a different place culturally. As MLC grew and developed, most member systems developed more formation elements, and now most are developing formal internal formation programs. Providence Health & Services designed the Providence Leadership Formation program, which is modeled on MLC and specifically designed for the next tier of leaders in the organization. Each member system strives to integrate the MLC program into its internal intrasystem formation to ensure a common language and to strengthen its ability to support a common culture of ministry leadership formation. The diversity among member systems provides for a rich reservoir of experiences from which to draw in designing and refining intersystem formation models. This wide breadth of placement along the continuum of intrasystem formation initiatives and experience also poses challenges to intersystem collaborative work because each system has distinct needs, readiness levels, and resources related to formation initiatives.

A foundational assumption at the onset of our MLC system integration work was that a clear boundary lies between the MLC program and each system's organizational hierarchy and infrastructure. While each system shares the common ground of serving Catholic Health Care and therefore participates in the ongoing revelation of what it means to operationalize the healing ministry of Jesus in the world of today, every system also has a distinct culture, organizational structure, and strategy. We recognize this diversity as an asset to the formation of leaders across the spectrum, and also

> A foundational assumption at the onset of our MLC system integration work was that a clear boundary lies between the MLC program and each system's organizational hierarchy and internal infrastructure.

respectfully look to each system's internal resources to support its leader participants in the program and to do the ongoing work of providing the specific context of the MLC formation experience to their organizational reality. A review of our history with system integration initiatives underscores our development; it also demonstrates how our technological platforms introduced a significant infrastructure that advanced integration initiatives more successfully. Equally important, and belied by a look at our historical journey, is the recognition that as each year passed, member systems began to build a critical mass of leaders with experience of MLC within their systems, which appropriately introduced the need and opportunity to address intrasystem mission integration differently, as well as to be attentive to ongoing formation needs of these leaders.

Historical Perspectives
on Intersystem Integration

The history of intersystem initiatives has been woven into our MLC design from the beginning in 2005. The inauguration of MLC included asking each system to identify an internal coordinator, whom we referred to as a "point person." The role of the point person was to serve as a liaison between MLC and the system. The point persons maintained a list of participants, distributed materials provided by MLC to participants and affiliated parties within their system, provided the names of future participants, and generally managed administrative functions. Each system selected and appointed their own point persons, who varied in title by system anywhere from vice presidents of mission integration to executive assistants. MLC provided each system point person with key documents and guidelines for dialogue partners, establishing from the beginning a consistent integration platform across systems. At this point a top-tier of executive leaders attended MLC, which eliminated the need for clear role expectations and participant selection criteria. The assumption generally in place across member systems was that established mission leaders would accompany participants and serve as dialogue partners. Because the program had just begun, knowledge about creating on-site internal systems and structures to support participants in off-site formation had not yet matured.

In 2007, the MLC board of directors, with two years of MLC experience, began sensing the value of the intersystem focus on leadership formation and articulated a need to adopt a common understanding of "integration." Integration was defined as "a process that encourages and enables MLC participants to competently incorporate their enhanced mission-related working knowledge and skills in the operation and governance of the ministries for which they are responsible." A clear understanding had emerged from the MLC experiment that intentional focus on the application of knowledge and skills by participants was necessary to drive intrasystem transformation, so much so that a "process to encourage and enable" such integration was started. In response to this identified need, MLC convened an intersystem formation focus group that identified four areas for further study: (1) a review of the structural elements of comprehensive formation programs, (2) the appropriate content of system formation programming, (3) the identification of formation facilitators and presenters, and (4) the use of a technology platform to support communication and collaboration.

The emphasis on integration began to shift from a focus on participant support to a broader consideration of intra- and inter-system formation programs and initiatives. With this subtle shift, there was a dovetailing of intra- and intersystem initiatives, which was hinged and fostered by the MLC program experience.

Three results emerged from this group. First, from an *intrasystem* perspective, member systems were recognizing the value in the MLC formation program and were seeking ways to leverage the MLC experience to enhance or develop additional formation opportunities within systems. Toward that end, a clear articulation of the key structural elements and the appropriate content of successful ministry leadership formation was named as essential. Second, from an *intersystem* perspective, there was the dawning of the idea that shared learning and experience could benefit the whole. The identification and compilation of seasoned formation facilitators and presenters for use among the systems was identified as a beneficial intersystem undertaking. And third, there was recognition that MLC's ability to *communicate and foster collaboration*, among participants and systems, would best occur via technology. In a few years, the emphasis on integration began to shift from a sole focus on participant support to a broader consideration of the possibilities inherent in intra- and intersystem formation programs and initiatives. With this subtle shift, there was a dovetailing of intra- and intersystem initiatives, which was hinged and fostered by the MLC program experience.

Shared Resources and Cooperation

MLC, seeking actionable intersystem formation initiatives based on the focus group's recommendations, conducted intrasystem surveys and interviews in 2009 to better assess and understand system needs. Sorting through the diversity of member systems and the variation in intrasystem systems and structures, MLC formed an Intersystem Formation Task Force and began very focused work on intersystem integration. The focus at this point centered on cooperation between systems and shared-practice learning. We simultaneously installed our first web platform, which served as the essential receptacle for further advancing intersystem cooperation and resource sharing. Toward that end, the Intersystem Formation Task Force, comprising members from all member systems, developed a comprehensive information center that includes:

- lists of the components of formation programs at all levels of the systems;

- outlines of the current common formation practices within systems;

- a compilation of existing system ministry leadership competencies and accountability structures;

- an articulation of a business case underscoring value and the operational benefit of MLC investment;

- a database of national formation presenters and facilitators; and

- a library of shared online resources to support participants, the alumni, and the system formation team.

The significant contributions of the our Intersystem Formation Task Force greatly increased cooperation between the systems and created a comprehensive information center of shared resources, which has benefited individual systems and promoted model practices among all member systems. We currently continue to support cooperation in system integration initiatives via this web platform, including a resource sharing library and the Action|Feedback process, which provides practical experience for participant's ongoing formation and valuable insights that inform strategic inter- and intrasystem initiatives. Additionally, Qualtrix, online survey software, provides relevant assessment data and tools for use in identifying and prioritizing intersystem initiatives, as well as a means for measuring participant and organizational development. And our integration efforts extend to alumni reunion and international cohorts, which provide avenues for demonstrating the value of ongoing formation around relevant and timely concerns as a means for continued and enhanced intersystem formation.

Three Distinct Concerns of Intersystem Integration

As the number of participants and alumni began to grow, there emerged greater need to address three key areas of concern to system integration:

- clear systems and structures outlining the criteria for the selection, ongoing support, and expectations of MLC participants;

- allocation of appropriate resources to support formal formation initiatives within member systems, including MLC, as well as intrasystem formation initiatives; and

- methods for not only sharing resources but, in the rapidly changing environment of health care and Catholic Health Care governance and sponsorship, developing authentic capacity for intersystem collaboration.

The burgeoning efforts in system integration were augmented by the practical experience of individual participants and the growing capacity of organizations to use a common language and to influence strategic and tactical decisions within systems. Our journey of integration highlighted a few learnings and some underdeveloped pockets of influence. MLC and our member systems assumed that formal mission leaders within systems would serve as companions to executives participating in MLC. However, the role and responsibility of mission leadership in relation to MLC was not necessarily overtly or consistently acknowledged or structured into job expectations within systems. This yielded inconsistent practices of support for participants and insufficient knowledge of MLC by many of these key people. Subsequently, identification of key formation elements within systems, such as succession planning, executive development, and organizational development initiatives, further creates questions of intrasystem formation support roles beyond mission, such as human resources.

Going forward it is critical that systems identify key intrasystem resources; in addition, they must leverage our essential partnership and ensure that these key leaders' roles are grounded in a consistent and comprehensive understanding of MLC and system expectations. This sort of grounding could take the form of a formal orientation or of a "form the formers" program in which MLC or member systems provide skills, knowledge, and facilitation training to support the resources dedicated to supporting and advancing intrasystem formation integration.

Additionally, we are learning that the very nature of intrasystem mission leadership roles is evolving and changing in relation to the MLC program. As executives grow in their ability to articulate and integrate the twelve foundational concerns, they start to function as integrated mission leaders themselves. Therefore, there is a distinct shift in the expectations of formal mission integration leaders and an emerging need to clarify the emerging priorities for these key roles within a ministry. Each system is distinct and within each system there are distinct subcultures all united under one mission. The work of deeply connecting these subcultures and strengthening their understanding of their local and larger system identity is important in intrasystem mission leadership. Subsequently, to link that system-specific identity and cultural story to the larger meta-story of Catholic Health Care, the systems partner with MLC. Through an approach to the twelve foundational concerns and with the accountability of Action|Feedback tailored to and practiced within particular cultural and operational realities, the MLC program begins the work of integrating a broader Catholic Health Care identity to the lived reality in very local and particular settings. Leaders become significant meaning-makers and culture-bearers within the systems in which they serve. They, in a very integrated way, become the modern face of mission leadership, dissolving the sense that there are mission people and business people and that they do not overlap, as well as the idea of formal mission people and the sisters as the only bearers of the Catholic identity. They are mission-driven business leaders. However, for formal mission leaders there remains distinct and important work in ongoing formation and in the facilitation of intrasystem formation that leavens larger organizational transformation.

The distinct nature of each member system and its development as a system in relation to intrasystem formation programs further challenges the work of comprehensive system integration work.

Future Horizons for Ongoing Cooperation and Collaboration

Future focus on successful integration rests on an articulation and establishment of dedicated internal resources committed to maximizing and leveraging the significant investment of participants and systems in MLC. Another key learning from our intersystem integration work is that as we focus on cooperation and shared resources, we must maintain a balance between integration as the support of the active and transitioned participant and as the system-wide impact and implications of the MLC experience on whole organizational cultures and practices. It is imperative in such an iterative and dialogic paradigm to continually examine and revise systems and structures to suit the changing dynamic. To achieve this balanced approach to integration, we recognize that point persons are essential in systems, but their role can no longer simply be that of an administrative liaison to an off-site formation experience. Internal resources will better serve the larger and broader MLC objectives of building and sustaining ministry leaders of the future, when system integration liaisons will serve as a system-wide strategic partners who are accountable for guiding and shaping intrasystem formation initiatives. These system leaders bring the knowledge and experience necessary to influence and guide the innovative collaborative initiatives facing all member systems into relationship with MLC staff and with one another as system counterparts. Such influence drives intrasystem integration and has the potential to guide the meta-story of Catholic Health Care in innovative and creative directions.

The formation experience requires that it function on the individual and organizational levels. Our approach to system integration includes a sensitivity to the fact that our system partners, mission and formation leaders, stand within and outside their organizations. They are prophetic voices and visionary flame-bearers of the tradition. In this way, they are of the organization but not fully in the organization. Community provides a network of peers from which to draw strength and perspective and is a significant need, particularly at this point in Catholic Health Care. The tradition, and certainly the founding religious orders, modeled working communally, in cooperation and collaboration. These examples laid a roadmap for approaches to our system integration work. Our approach leads us to understand that creativity develops within community and that the formation process is communal because by its very nature it situates the individual leaders within collective conversations. We intuitively know that this understanding will hold true for our formation integration teams going forward as well. Approaching our work of intra- and intersystem integration within a community of practice, we believe, will serve well in both integration and the formation program. As in the old adage, we are better together than we are alone.

Current Efforts in Strengthening Collaboration

In 2012, MLC formed a Formation Integration Team (FIT). Drawing from our refreshed understanding of approaches to system integration and reiterating our commitment to cooperation and collaboration, we identified that in system integration our essential partnership is with the system-level persons with the

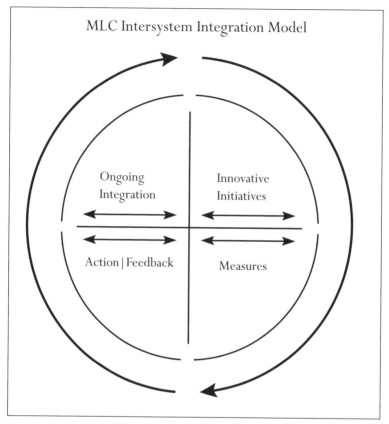

Figure 9.2 Four focuses of the Formation Integration Team (FIT)

accountability to drive formation integration within their systems. FIT begins the work of building a collaboration that supports doing formation across systems and of developing model practices and template approaches to shared concerns using the best thinking and a common articulation of a Catholic Health Care ethos. If this sort of intersystem collaboration happens, just as the intersystem formation experience of the program informs and enriches the participant experience, systems will have the opportunity to inform and enrich the whole community of Catholic Health Care and to consider a common way in which the tradition is developing in light of its founding revelation and contemporary cultural challenges. The FIT charter echoes our original articulated goals based on intersystem initiatives, which include three components:

- *consultation* to support MLC alumni and participants;

- *coordination* of resources to support and enhance intrasystem formation initiatives; and

- *facilitation* of intersystem collegiality and collaboration.

We developed a diagram to illustrate how intersystem integration can function most effectively and how it requires that integration be addressed through the partnership of MLC and each member system. (See figure 9.2.) This diagram is divided into four quadrants. The arrow within each quadrant illustrates that each member system finds itself at a different place along the continuum of integration.

"Ongoing integration" references the basic systems and structures necessary to strategically align and tactically integrate the MLC experience as a member system. It speaks specifically to the administrative functions of record-keeping, communication, and resources, and to the basic participant support of dialogue partners, Action|Feedback, and alumni and local cohort management. It also extends the strategic alignment of MLC to succession planning, executive development, and organizational development.

"Innovative initiatives" references the creative and emerging shared work between the member systems. It speaks specifically to areas of shared interest and concern where concerted and coordinated collaborative work would yield benefit for all systems. Current areas of concern and focus related to innovative initiatives are identified as physician leadership development and formation, formal reporting mechanisms to account for fidelity to Catholic identity with ecclesial partners and sponsor or governance bodies, and models for effective engagement with partners and affiliates who are not Catholic.

"Measures" references the ongoing value and importance of effective qualitative and quantitative measures in demonstrating the value and developmental advances for individuals and organizations related to the MLC experience. System integration will most effectively tell its story when it can articulate the means to measure and assess cultural transformation. We see this as a key component of system integration.

"Action|Feedback" references the bridge we have built directly between the program and the systems. Participants practice the articulation and integration of the twelve foundational concerns in the setting of their specific ministries. These opportunities become formation experiences for the recipients of Action|Feedback. An opportunity to harness and shape larger transformation in the organization of the culture exists in understanding and leveraging the learning of Action|Feedback. It is a critical part of system integration.

Emerging Realities Related to System Integration

System integration has evolved to a place where we must rely on our member systems to guide and facilitate the organizational leveraging of not only individual participant's formation experience but also the broader ministry's knowledge regarding the effective ministry leadership formation gained from the essential partnership of the program. Just as at its inception our approach included a teaching but did not have an infrastructure to support and account for participant's turning their formational experience into working knowledge, so too was system integration infrastructure loosely defined by MLC. It also varied significantly from system and system. With the development of the website and the development of Action|Feedback, participant accountability increased and the active and effective practice of articulation and integration of these concerns into organizational life began to occur. This articulation is an active catalyst to intrasystem formation and cultural development which now can be leveraged, supported, directed, and aligned systematically within systems. Such a commitment and engagement will deepen the value and success of the core commitment to have all members of a system become more deeply aligned with the organizational mission, vision, and values.

Catholic Health Care is traditionally quite isolationist. We are learning to find the common ground, of which ministry leadership formation is part, and to serve as support to one another in order to form a professional and ministerial perspective and navigate the competitive boundaries system to system. It is quite remarkable to see the shared concern and camaraderie begin to form among the Formation Integration Team. We identify this as a ripe opportunity to form community and model a way of working in cooperation and collaboration, which has been an essential dynamic of the tradition.

As the work of continuing to support and direct intersystem integration occurs, we will explore expanding to include new member systems who would benefit from learning system integration. We continue to follow the lead of discovery that grows from the dynamic partnership that we have with individual participants and their representative systems. This path has led us to current practices; and the scoped work of system integration remains within known paradigms, but the horizon of effective and relevant inter- and intrasystem formation is leading to uncharted territory wild with creative opportunity. We are on unpaved roads, a place where the tradition and our founding sisters frequently found themselves. Inspired and encouraged by the same founding revelation, we seek to advance the tradition as our original sponsors did, as a community, working collaboratively in service to the common good.

The Future of Leadership Formation

Laurence J. O'Connell and John Shea

The future of leadership formation is dependent on who wants it to happen and how serious they are in committing resources to accomplish it. As the introduction pointed out, the Ministry Leadership Center was conceived and founded by the collaborative efforts of bishops, sponsors, and system CEOs. The key stakeholders wanted it to happen; and since MLC's founding, the six sponsoring systems have given the Center their unequivocal financial and emotional support. It is this level of uncompromising commitment that makes possible creative programming and ensures the engaged participation of leaders. As organizational literature continually asserts, top-down modeling by the most senior leaders is crucial to successful organizational initiatives.

> The future of leadership formation is dependent on who wants it to happen and how serious they are in committing resources to accomplish it.

Once the Ministry Leadership Formation Program was established, holding the goals of the program firmly in mind and being attentive to emerging possibilities shaped its subsequent development. Through constant questioning, we uncovered new paths and expanded horizons. In an earlier article, "Ministry Leadership Formation: Engaging with Leaders," we listed questions that were already opening up future directions for our program.[1]

We grouped them into questions about organizational positioning and about program refinement. We assume that other programs would benefit from a similar set of questions.

Organizational Positioning

- How does the organization choose participants?

- How is the organizational impact of ministry leadership formation assessed?

- After leaders have finished the program, how should ongoing formation be conducted?

- How do board and associate formation align with ministry leadership formation?

- How does ministry leadership formation complement other leadership development programs?

Program Refinement

- What is the most relevant content in each of the twelve areas?

- Who are the most effective presenters and facilitators?

- How can program, participants, and organizational impact be more effectively evaluated?

- How are the off-site sessions integrated into on-site ministry leadership opportunities?

- What type of formational support is needed between sessions and how is it delivered?

- How are the special requests—for example, more sensitivity to diversity issues—of individual participants and systems honored?

As we look at this list today, we realize that we have addressed and continue to address these questions. The list has naturally grown because time brings new possibilities and because supplying even partial answers inevitably leads to more questions and expanded thinking. For instance:

- How is sponsor formation connected to board, leader, and associate formation?

- When the organization hires and promotes, what weight is given to excellence in articulating and integrating Catholic identity?

- How does the organization support and reward participation in the program?

- Have standardized formation assessment tools been developed and used?

- Can mission leaders or chaplaincy take on the tasks of board, leader, and associate formation?

- How do leaders who have participated in the MLC program understand and relate to those who have not participated?

These questions target directly the activity of ministry formation in its programmatic form and organizational context.

But since leadership formation is intrinsically linked to the larger issues of health care in general and Catholic Health Care in particular, almost everything that is occurring has ramifications for ministry formation:

- How is ministry formation negotiated when Catholic systems merge, affiliate, and partner with non-Catholic systems?

- How do for-profit entities within Catholic systems affect Catholic identity and mission?

- What are the ministry formation implications as Catholic Health Care develops different relations with physicians?

- How do public policy initiatives like the Affordable Care Act facilitate or threaten Catholic identity and mission?

- How do the theological perspectives and public policy positions of individual bishops affect Catholic Health Care?

- How do we follow and support leaders who have gone through the formation process as they move from position to position and even from system to system?

But, on the whole, determining today what key questions to ask, prioritize, and begin to answer is probably the most immediate and reliable way into tomorrow.

Those with more complete information and a keener appreciation of what trends will dominate in the near term could sharpen these questions and add others. But, on the whole, determining today what key questions to ask, prioritize, and begin to answer is probably the most immediate and reliable way into tomorrow. As Peter Drucker commented, "Strategic planning does not deal with future decisions. It deals with the futurity of present decisions."[2]

"Will Whatever We Do Be Enough?"

But simply supplying a practical checklist of critical questions surrounding approaches to the future of ministry leadership formation does not address important underlying concerns. For example, there is often a nagging doubt that surrounds the concrete tasks of ministry leadership formation and that haunts the enterprise from within: "Will whatever we do be enough?" An atmosphere of hesitancy enters the efforts.

This type of vacillation often occurs when the transition from one form of identity and mission to another form of identity and mission involves major discontinuities; and that is often the case with contemporary Catholic Health Care. Whatever form Catholic Health Care takes in the future, it will be significantly different from what it has been in the immediate past. Therefore, this inner wavering about the feasibility of continuing the tradition through leadership formation is a tempting perspective.

- Too much discontinuity is just another name for loss. The mind entertains the voices of larger cultural forces that predict demise.

- Leadership formation is too little too late. It won't work.

- Western history is evolving from religious institutions into secular enterprises and soon all faith-based organizations will fade.

- Conscience clauses will push Catholic social organizations out of business.

- Some Catholic systems will sell and set up foundations; others will slowly lose their Catholic sensibility.

- In the popular mind Catholic Health Care is going to be reduced to the medical procedures it won't do.

- Big and impersonal health care systems will undercut Catholic values; so even if Catholic Health Care stays around, it will be in name only.

- It is just not possible for Catholic Health Care to survive the loss of the nuns.

- It's a different age; the best advice is to forget the past and get on with the future.

- Leaders are interested in leading and retiring, but not in continuing a tradition.

The message of these voices of doubt suggests that there are too many forces—legal, structural, theological, attitudinal—lined up against ministry leadership formation to believe that it can facilitate and resource a new and future form of Catholic Health Care.

Of course, a rational approach to this type of eroding doubt is to line up the suppositions of this cultural barrage and whittle them down, one by one. Each is capable of being refuted. But since they are assumptions people work from rather than conclusions that have been argued, disproving them does not have the effect of eliminating them. Their persuasiveness comes neither from inner logic nor empirical data, so pointing out logical inconsistencies or providing disconfirming data does little to eliminate these doubts that are usually non-rational, if not indeed irrational.

These voices of doubt persist because they sing a song that our finite existence knows only too well. They create a consciousness that connects and unleashes the emotional power of inevitable loss against which we feel helpless. The single message of the multiple voices is: "All cultural forms perish; and the time of Catholic Health Care in America is over. All efforts to sustain it are futile." Once this enervating consciousness captures us, it slows the quickness of our mind, saps the resoluteness of our will, and dulls the creativity of our spirit. The only question we now ask ourselves is: "Why have we given ourselves to what destiny has decreed is over?" (Note well: this question does not appear on the questions listed earlier.) In this emotionally swamped situation, our only hope is to form a different consciousness that can include loss even as it transcends it in action.

> The message of these voices of doubt suggests that there are too many forces—legal, structural, attitudinal—lined up against leadership formation.

The Gift of the Founding Sisters

More than two decades ago Vaclav Havel, then president of Czecho-slovakia, reflected on hope.

> *Hope is not the same thing as optimism. . . . It is not the conviction that something will turn out well, but the certainty that something makes sense regardless of how it turns out. Hope, in this deep and powerful sense, is not the same as joy that things are going well, or willingness to invest in enterprises that are obviously headed for*

early success, but rather an ability to work for something because it is good, not just because it stands a chance to succeed. [This type of hope] gives us the strength to live and continually try new things, even in conditions that seem hopeless.[3]

The consciousness Havel describes is also captured in a folk tale. A man is walking down a road and sees a very elderly couple planting a tree. He says to them, "Why do you do this? You will never know if the tree grows or perishes; and you will never know the results of your labor." The woman responds, "The good is enough." We suspect the founding sisters of Catholic Health Care in America would agree with Havel's rendition of hope as well as nod and smile at this folktale.[4]

The founding sisters are often portrayed as women of moral virtue. They were dedicated to the needs of the poor even as they were solicitous of the rich, personally humble yet entrepreneurial for their ministries, compassionate to all but able to confront wrongdoing, resolute yet open to accommodations, admitting the strength of sin but believing in repentance, searching out people of good will yet demanding good intentions from anyone with whom they associated. This mosaic of virtues (and many more could be included) was developed in the interaction of deep faith and the harsh and demanding realities of caring for the sick. When we look back to founders, we focus on these virtues and realize they transcend time and are needed by ministry leaders today.

Yet virtues were not the whole picture. The sisters were theological creatures to their core. Their human virtues were grounded in faith convictions and renewed in spiritual practices that supported and purified whatever natural gifts they had. One of these key faith convictions had to do with the active presence of God. They believed the divine spirit animated human life and called out to those who could hear to cooperate in bringing about a better world. They had heard this call and had been taught to hear it again and again. Discernment, the skill of listening and responding to the lure of God in rough and tumble situations, was built into their being. They were committed to doing God's will.

But they were not committed to their rendition of how things would turn out as they worked to do God's will. The good had to be engaged without hesitation and without reserve. But the outcome was in God's hand. They lived with complete commitment to the good and complete openness to what that commitment would bring about.

We believe that this understanding of hope should be retrieved from the Catholic Health Care tradition and infused into all formation efforts.

When it brought about what they assessed as positive results, they gave thanks to God, the ultimate author. When it failed to achieve what they assessed as positive results, they suffered the humbling of their expectations and began to look for the good in what they perceived as the less-than-good results. The adventure of world transformation did not end when an old form did not survive or an expected form did not materialize.

This consciousness of action for the good without knowing the outcome was most evident in the tension between glaring need and insufficient resources. When the sisters confronted a human need that had to be addressed but did not have the resources to address it, they often forged ahead and did what they could. They always suspected that God was present in the need and calling out to those who could hear. So once they acted, resources would arrive to help them better the situation. Once again, their response was predictable. If resources did arrive, they thanked God. (The oral histories of religious congregations of women are rife with stories of deep pockets arriving in the nick of time.) If resources did not arrive, they did what they could. The work was good in itself and it had to be undertaken.

We believe that this understanding of hope should be retrieved from the Catholic Health Care tradition and infused into all formation efforts. It combines a commitment to articulating and integrating the twelve foundational concerns with openness to what that commitment will produce and where that commitment will lead. This consciousness is not a wait and see approach. It admits to not knowing the final future, but it cultivates the immediate work and multiple short-term goals. It is attuned to the Spirit of what has to be done and cooperates fully with it; and in the process it shapes and reshapes contemporary forms that will embody it. When this type of hope informs our consciousness, it generates fierce attention, creative action, and resilient response. These are the virtues that are suited for the long haul of Catholic Health Care's transition into its next future.

Notes

1. Laurence J. O'Connell and John Shea, "Ministry Leadership Formation: Engaging with Leaders," *Health Progress*, September-October 2009.

2. Peter F. Drucker, *Management: Tasks, Responsibilities, Practices* (London: Routledge, 2011), 119.

3. Vaclav Havel, *Disturbing the Peace: A Conversation with Karel Hvizdala*, trans. Paul Wilson (New York: Vintage, 1990), chap. 5, "The Politics of Hope."

4. See Barbara Mann Wall, *Unlikely Entrepreneurs* (Columbus: Ohio State University Press, 2005).

Appendices

Session Evaluation Form

*This is an example of a Session Evaluation Form,
in this case for the Vocation session.*

1. Thinking of all the presentations, materials, and discussions about identifying, adopting, and enhancing the vocational attitude toward work, how would you rate your own learning level?

| 1 | 2 | 3 | 4 | 5 | 6 | 7 | 8 | 9 | 10 |

Did not really learn much　　　　　　　　　　　**Learned a great deal**

2. In understanding the basic formational and educational approach of the program, how helpful was the section the Triangle?

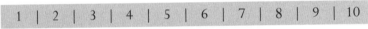

| 1 | 2 | 3 | 4 | 5 | 6 | 7 | 8 | 9 | 10 |

Not at all helpful　　　　　　　　　　　**Very helpful**

3. In improving your working knowledge and skills on Vocation, how helpful was the section on job, career, and calling?

| 1 | 2 | 3 | 4 | 5 | 6 | 7 | 8 | 9 | 10 |

Not at all helpful　　　　　　　　　　　**Very helpful**

4. In improving your working knowledge and skills on Vocation, how helpful was the section of Vocation as meaningful work?

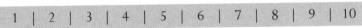

| 1 | 2 | 3 | 4 | 5 | 6 | 7 | 8 | 9 | 10 |

Not at all helpful　　　　　　　　　　　**Very helpful**

5. In improving your working knowledge and skills on Vocation, how helpful was the section on why Vocation is important?

| 1 | 2 | 3 | 4 | 5 | 6 | 7 | 8 | 9 | 10 |

Not at all helpful   Very helpful

6. In improving your working knowledge and skills on Vocation, how helpful was the section on the Catholic tradition: Universal Call and Vocational Community?

| 1 | 2 | 3 | 4 | 5 | 6 | 7 | 8 | 9 | 10 |

Not at all helpful   Very helpful

7. In improving your working knowledge and skills on Vocation, how helpful was the section on Five Stories of Adopting a Vocational Attitude?

| 1 | 2 | 3 | 4 | 5 | 6 | 7 | 8 | 9 | 10 |

Not at all helpful   Very helpful

8. In improving your working knowledge and skills on Vocation, how helpful was the section on emphasizing enjoyment and excellence?

| 1 | 2 | 3 | 4 | 5 | 6 | 7 | 8 | 9 | 10 |

Not at all helpful   Very helpful

9. In improving your working knowledge and skills on Vocation, how helpful was the section on investing attention?

| 1 | 2 | 3 | 4 | 5 | 6 | 7 | 8 | 9 | 10 |

Not at all helpful   Very helpful

10. In improving your working knowledge and skills on Vocation, how helpful was the section on remembering larger purposes?

| 1 | 2 | 3 | 4 | 5 | 6 | 7 | 8 | 9 | 10 |

Not at all helpful   Very helpful

11. In improving your working knowledge and skills on Vocation, how helpful was the section on developing a vocational ear and voice?

| 1 | 2 | 3 | 4 | 5 | 6 | 7 | 8 | 9 | 10 |

Not at all helpful   Very helpful

12. How well do you think the section on Action|Feedback prepared you to do something at home base?

| 1 | 2 | 3 | 4 | 5 | 6 | 7 | 8 | 9 | 10 |

Not at all helpful   Very helpful

13. Please rate your honest desire to participate in the next session of this program?

| 1 | 2 | 3 | 4 | 5 | 6 | 7 | 8 | 9 | 10 |

Not interested   Very interested

14. Overall, what was the most significant learning for you personally?

15. General comments and observations:

Presenter Form

This form is sent to all presenters.

The Ministry Leadership Formation Program

The Ministry Leadership Center (MLC) was created by five Catholic Health Care systems that have health care ministries in California—St. Joseph Health, Providence Health & Services, Dignity Health (formerly Catholic Healthcare West), SCL Health System (formerly Sisters of Charity of Leavenworth), and Daughters of Charity. Recently a sixth system, PeaceHealth, has joined the five founding systems. The purpose of MLC is to provide senior leaders with the working knowledge and skills that are necessary to lead the mission and ministry of Catholic Health Care.

To do this, MLC has designed a three-year Ministry Leadership Formation Program (MLFP). The first year focuses on the identity of leaders in Catholic Health Care.

> *As leaders in Catholic Health Care, we understand ourselves as (1) called to this work (2) in the context of a ministerial tradition that ultimately takes its inspiration and direction from the healing mission of Jesus. As part of this tradition, (3) we are committed personally and professionally to the spiritually grounded values (4) that guide our work in responding to human suffering.*

The second and third year focus on the work of leaders in Catholic Health Care.

> *As leaders in Catholic Health Care, we work (5) to integrate core values into organizational structures, policies, and behaviors; (6) to link discernment to strategic decision-making, innovation, and*

team composition; (7) to incorporate the Catholic social tradition into organizational life and mission; (8) to develop and ensure accountability for ethical policies, practices, and behaviors in our clinical settings; (9) to develop and ensure accountability for ethical policies, practices, and behaviors in our organizational relationships; (10) to bring the benefits of health care to the poorest and most vulnerable members of our society; (11) to respect and attend to the whole person of patients, physicians, associates, and volunteers; (12) and to work collaboratively with Church authorities and agencies.

Over the three-year period, there are twelve two-day sessions that provide the working knowledge and skills in these mission areas of Catholic Health Care leadership.

The Triangle of Catholic tradition, cultural information, and individual and communal experience is the framework for developing the working knowledge and skills in these twelve areas.

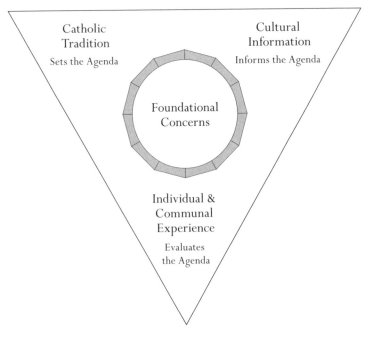

Catholic
Tradition
Sets the Agenda

Cultural
Information
Informs the Agenda

Foundational
Concerns

Individual &
Communal
Experience
Evaluates
the Agenda

This framework takes seriously the fact that the Catholic Health Care tradition always interfaces with cultural information, and that tradition and culture both influence and are critiqued by individual and communal experience. When all three points of the Triangle are consciously brought into dialogue, tradition is honored and brought forward, culture is acknowledged and engaged, and personal experience is both informed and allowed its own distinctive voice. In shorthand, the tradition sets the agenda; the culture informs the agenda; individual and communal experience evaluates the agenda.

The Role of Presenters

The presenters, in dialogue with the program director and the staff, are asked to: (1) suggest pre-session content for input/ exercises; (2) develop an approach to their topic that is interactive and divided into sections; and (3) develop exercises and materials that participants could use in their work settings, in particular with their management teams.

Pre-Session Requirements

There are always pre-session requirements. Recently, we have moved to expecting participants to work with input/exercises. These are papers, two to five pages long, that supply some critical and relevant content on the session topic and an exercise that helps them integrate that content. An example would be an input that describes both a dissonant and a resonant leader and an exercise question directed at their experience of both a dissonant and resonant leader and what impact it had on them. The results of this exercise are discussed with when the group comes together.

Interactive and Sectioned

Our two-day sessions are interactive. Presenters are asked to keep presentations to thirty minutes and provide questions that participants can use in groups of five (or whatever size would be best) to process the material and connect it to some aspect of their work situations and health care issues in general.

Our day-and-a-half sessions are also broken down into sections. For example, the session on Catholic social teaching had sections that focused on using Catholic social principles to vet forces affecting health care, fashioning Catholic social principles into a leadership vision, connecting Catholic social concern with all people of good will, and so on. This sectioning provides clarity to the content of each of the twelve mission areas and gives the program designers a way of knowing what sections are most helpful.

Using What Has Been Learned

The participants are also asked to pass along in one way or another some of what they learned at their day-and-a-half session. Therefore, presenters are asked to make recommendations on how they might do this. This would include anything from a short teaching module to instructions on how to integrate the material into some ongoing aspect of their work environment. The idea is for the participants to integrate what they have learned into their leadership activities. They report back what they have done in this area in an Action|Feedback forum.

System Expectations for Dialogue Partners

This is an example of a system adaptation of dialogue partner expectations.

Providence Health & Services

Purpose

Dialogue partners assist Ministry Leadership Center (MLC) participants in the articulation and integration of the MLC learnings. The dialogue partner raises questions or concerns and explores ideas for self-awareness and personal and professional formation.

Criteria

An understanding of Catholic Health Care ministry and how mission is integrated at Providence Health & Services as well as skills in active listening and reflection are required.

Responsibilities

The dialogue partner is expected to be available to meet or speak with the MLC participant once a month for approximately sixty minutes. They must be willing to read MLC materials before the dialogue, which should take approximately four hours per quarter. And they must be committed to participating for one year and possibly for the full three-year program.

Key Learnings to Date

The process of dialoguing is an enrichment process for both the MLC participant and the dialogue partner. It is an opportunity to get to know each other at a different level, developing a relationship of trust within a sacred space. It is a process to assist MLC participants and dialogue partners to have conversations about many aspects of their life.

Tips

It is helpful to be located at the same site as the participant to facilitate face-to-face meetings. The partner can be someone inside or outside participant's discipline. The monthly meetings should be scheduled; if circumstances require change, reschedule the meeting rather than canceling it

Selection Process

After the first MLC session, names of past and current MLC dialogue partners will be distributed via email to the group participants (a partner does not have to be selected from this list). The MLC participant identifies and contacts a potential partner, describes the purpose and responsibilities of the role and the key learnings to date, and invites the person to serve in this role.

Support

After all dialogue partners are selected, they are invited to participate in an orientation teleconference hosted by the Providence Health & Services Mission Leadership Department. MLC session summaries and monthly reflection papers are forwarded to the dialogue partners. The Providence Health & Services dialogue partners are coordinated by Susan Keyes, System Manager, Ministry Leadership Formation, who is the Point Person with MLC.

One-Page Reflection Paper

This is an example of one-page reflection paper.

Vocational Leaders Engage Challenges

Some time back, I attended a reception that honored the college-age winners of a city-wide art competition. An older artist addressed the winners. His first words were, "If you pursue the vocation of an artist in our society, here are some of the challenges you will face."

He didn't sugarcoat it; and he didn't paint it so grim that he "thinned the crowd" of potential artists. He just laid it out as he saw it.

But you could see that he was into the artistic, cultural, and financial challenges. These were not unfortunate situations that were happening to him and that he was complaining about. They were factors he engaged, eager for the opportunities they provided him. They defined who he was and what his work was about.

At our Vocation session, we explored a number of ways that the vocational sense of leadership in Catholic Health Care could be enhanced. Perhaps the perspective and attitude of this artist could enrich and direct our conversation.

When Catholic Health Care leaders see their work as a vocation, they also simultaneously sense that the path ahead will not be completely smooth. There will be obstacles, difficulties that come with the territory of leading the ministry of Catholic Health Care: "Given that this is who we are as Catholic Health Care, and given that this is the society in which we live, and given that this is where medicine is at, these difficulties are inevitable." In a sense,

Catholic Health Care co-creates its difficulties. The difficulties begin when we take a vocational stance: "This is who we are and this is what we are called to do."

Therefore, the vocational sense does not bemoan difficulties and wish they would go away. Rather, it turns them into challenges. Meeting these challenges is not only necessary to carry out the mission. It also is a way the vocational sense is strengthened and clarified. Catholic Health Care leaders get good at living with these challenges, become wise in their ways, engage their arguments, foresee their strategies, and persevere in what is possible. Vocational leaders become seasoned by the difficulties they turn into challenges and by the challenges they engage.

- Take some time and jot down a few of the ongoing challenges that come with the vocation of leading Catholic Health Care.

- Ask your dialogue partner or another person in the program what she or he thinks are some of the ongoing challenges that come with the vocation of leading Catholic Health Care.

Session Summary

This is an example of a session summary.

Whole Person Care

Whole Person Care primarily refers to how hospital staff and medical caregivers relate to patients, their families and loved ones. We will explore these relationships in another session. In our September sessions, we focused on the organizational context that models and supports whole person patient care. We addressed how leaders care for themselves and their people as they do the work that needs to be done: whole person worker care.

Brother Jim Zullo supplied a model of circles of support networks. The two inner circles—God and self-intimacy/soul mates—were non-negotiable. The outer circles were more variable. Then we used the model to analyze where we are receiving support and where we need more support.

With this analysis in place, the message of whole person worker care was stated: without support and self-intimacy, we are not able to manage stress and we become vulnerable to burnout or depression and the addictions.

We described stress as "a particular relationship between the person and the environment that is appraised by the person as taxing or exceeding his or her resources and endangering his or her well-being." If we do not manage this "appraised stress" well through careful attention and a number of different practices, we open ourselves to burnout.

Burnout looks like overwork, but at its core is a loss of our circles of support. The red flags of burnout are decreased energy, decreased self-esteem, output exceeding input, a sense of hopelessness, feeling trapped, a loss of idealism, cynicism and negativism, self-deprecation, putting yourself down, being TUBED—tired,used, bored, and envious, with a death wish—hopelessness. Burnout can lead to depression. Depression is best understood as a continuum ranging from wellness to illness. Jim also helped us understand how burnout makes us vulnerable to the addictions.

The way out of burnout is to reverse the path into burnout—nurture the center circles, hold on to your core purpose, and take care of your inner self and your significant relationships. Larry added to this understanding of whole person wellness by exploring the positive purpose of leisure and highlighting how it is crucial to the Catholic tradition, which sees the whole person as a balance of being and doing, work and leisure.

Following the lead of emotionally intelligent leadership, we emphasized self-knowledge as a way of self-care. We shared our work on the Leadership Identity Statement and what we learned about ourselves in doing that project. We also recognized that leaders have a complex relationship to the Catholic Health Care tradition—resonating with some of it, respecting some of it, and wanting some of it reviewed and changed.

Finally, we emphasized how these leadership dynamics of self-care are present in their people. In particular, we recognized how leaders must always overcome the distance between themselves and their people through listening and learning. We discussed how to prepare to listen as well as the actual practice of listening. We also suggested how leaders learn from their people and how they communicate to their people what they are learning. Becoming a listener and learner is an effective way to care for your people.

Pre-Session Input/Exercise

This is an example of a pre-session input/exercise.

Partnering with Catholic Social Teaching

Official Catholic teaching often positions Catholic Health Care within the Catholic social tradition. Therefore, Catholic social teaching (CST) should guide its organization and mission.

Principles

CST is often articulated in terms of core principles like human dignity and the common good and secondary principles that are derived from these core principles like reverence for life, such as participation and subsidiarity, solidarity, preferential option for the poor, right of association, and so on. The two core principles are constant and are rooted in theological convictions.

But the amount of secondary principles can change and increase because new situations have to be addressed in light of the core principles. For example, today many people want to spin the core principle of the common good into a secondary principle of diversity because diversity seems to be a path to the common good that is relevant to the contemporary situation.

Core and secondary principles are foundational. However, if they are to have an impact, they need to move from generality to specificity. Although secondary principles begin that process, they do not go far enough. The fact is that the teaching itself, as teaching, is never going to spell out solutions to the problems of particular situations. It will always be too general.

Always General

Read the witnesses, from popes to theologians to a committee from the United States National Conference of Catholic Bishops, on the generality of CST. (The emphasis in the quotations is ours.)

Catholic social teaching rarely if ever gets very concrete and specific.

—Dennis Doyle, *The Church Emerging from Vatican II* (Mystic, Conn.: Twenty-Third Publications, 1992).

[In Catholic social teaching] the question is always general; so is the response. Whatever the question, the answer is usually framed in a few general principles accompanied by several guidelines for programs consistent with the principles. For a universal teaching Church, this is the way it has to be, I suppose.

—William Byron, "The Future of Catholic Social Thought," *Catholic University Law Review* 4 (1993): 557.

Catholic teaching does not and cannot provide specific answers to many difficult and complex questions. However, it can offer direction and help shape the dialogue about what is a just and fair workplace and how workers participate in the decisions which affect them.

—United States Conference of Catholic Bishops, "A Fair and Just Work-place": Principles and Practices for Catholic Health Care.

Obviously a continuum exists from the more general, to the less general, to the less specific, to the more specific. Recall that the U.S. bishops distinguished between formal church teaching, universal moral principles, and application of these moral principles to particular issues. The bishops recognized that their application of principles involved prudential judgments that can be interpreted differently by people of good will and by Catholics within the same faith community.

—Charles E. Curran, *Catholic Social Teaching, 1891–Present* (Washington, D.C.: Georgetown University Press, 2002), 113.

The writings [Catholic social teaching] are attempts to speak to the broad audience of worldwide Catholicism and, even beyond the confines of the Catholic community, the global audience "all people of good will." Consequently, one finds in this teaching few specifics and many broad general statements. The teaching does not delve into the specifics of proposed solutions but functions more at the level of values and perspectives by which to frame discussion of a problem and understand what is at stake. These are not documents that will satisfy all the requirements of social ethics or public policy analysis; nor are they meant to do so.

—Kenneth R. Himes, O.F.M., *Modern Catholic Social Teaching: Commentaries and Interpretations* (Washington, D.C.: Georgetown University Press, 2004), 5.

Why?

Why will the teaching as teaching always remain general? According to Pope Paul VI, it is because of an essential tension between the universal and local that cannot be resolved by people on the universal level:

In the face of widely varying situations it is difficult for us to utter a unified message and to put forth a solution which has universal validity. Such is not our ambition, nor is it our mission. It is up to the Christian communities to analyze with objectivity the situation which is proper to their own country, to shed on it the light of the Gospel's unalterable words and to draw principles of reflection, norms of judgment and directives for action from the social teaching of the church.

—Paul VI, *Octogesima adveniens*, 4.

According to Pope John Paul II, it is because the people on the universal level lack the competence to make the connections to concrete situations:

The Church does not have technical revolutions to offer for the problem of underdevelopment as such, as Pope Paul VI already affirmed in his Encyclical. For the Church does not propose economic and political systems or programs, nor does she show preference for one or the other, provided that human dignity is properly respected and promoted, and provided she herself is allowed the room she needs to exercise her ministry in the world.

—John Paul II

Therefore, since the essential tension between the universal and local cannot be resolved by only one side, the universal, and since the universal is not, by definition, competent in local affairs, CST is not going to work unless it finds people who will embrace it, struggle with it, and implement it in specific situations.

Partner?

Leaders in Catholic Health Care are called to partner with CST to articulate and integrate it into concrete situations. They have what the people at the top who formulate the teaching do not have: the knowledge of concrete situations and the competency to influence them.

However, this partnering is a difficult undertaking. It is not a matter of simple compliance with norms. It requires a good deal of learning and discipline. Moving from general principles to specific situations entails imaginative and creative efforts.

Therefore, it is good at the outset to gauge how interested we are in taking on this project. Please rate your interest on the scale:

How interested are you in learning how to articulate and integrate CST into your leadership?

| 1 | 2 | 3 | 4 | 5 | 6 | 7 | 8 | 9 | 10 |

Not interested   **Very interested**

When we get together for our session, we will share our interest levels and the reasons for how we rated that interest.

Instructions for the Practice of Silence

This is an example of instructions for the practice of silence.

The very fact of taking time to be silent introduces balance into our lives. We are people who live with our consciousness in the outer world. From the time we wake until the time we go to bed, we are traveling into the territories of work and personal life. When we engage in silence—no matter what we do with that silent time—we naturally pull consciousness inside, take it out of the outer world, and allow it to rest. That alone brings an inclusiveness, a completeness, a wholeness.

Think of silence as a house with many rooms where there are a set of instructions for each room. We will enter many rooms in the course of our three-year program. In each room we will give a different set of instructions. But we are always free to do with the silence whatever we think is appropriate. The instructions are always suggestions. But they will introduce to some of the practices that our ancestors thought were important.

The instructions we want to attend to today are sometimes called Touch and Go. They acknowledge that we are people moving from a past through a present into a future. However, there is a way in which we carry the past into every present; and when we do, we are often not as fully present in the moment as we could be. A past happening preoccupies us. We are still chewing food that we have eaten.

The future can also impinge on the present in such a way that we are not as present in the moment as we could be. What we have to do tomorrow occupies our mind. So, in this story line, silence is a way for us to clear our minds of the past and future in order to be more fully where we are at—in the present moment. Be here now, as the slogan goes.

Therefore, in our silence today, we can acknowledge how our minds are holding on to the past by touching all those contents and letting them go. Do not push them out of the mind, for then they will still have a hold on us. They are our thoughts and we must respect them, even if we cannot in all cases love them. Letting them go shows that we are a little bit more than our minds.

We do the same things with future thoughts. We touch them and respect them. After all, they are things that need doing and are part of our responsibilities. But right now something else is afoot, and we need to be fully present to it. So we can let go of this future agenda. We will attend to it as it arrives. In short, do not worry about the future. The future will worry about itself.

You might want to try this inner activity during the silent time. It is a way of being more fully present to where you are. And we want that to be the case for the next day and a half.

Contributors

Andre L. Delbecq, DBA, served as the dean of the Business School at Santa Clara University for ten years. He currently serves as the McCarthy Professor of Management and Director for the Institute for Spirituality of Organizational Leadership at Santa Clara. He is the MLC Senior Fellow for Spirituality and Organizational Leadership.

Bill Fitzgerald, BA, MA, served as a technology director for over ten years, where he developed curriculum and training materials for youth and adults. Bill initiated and manages the Drupal in Education Group on http://groups.drupal.org and is active in various educational and open-sourced communities. He is the MLC Senior Fellow for Communities of Practice.

Sharyn Lee has over forty-five years of administrative experience in a variety of fields, including positions with General Electric, the Arizona State Legislature, and the University of California, Davis. She is the MLC Director of Administrative Services.

Elizabeth McCabe, BA, MALS, has worked in three formal ministries of the Church—Social Services, Education, and Health Care. Most recently, Elizabeth served in Providence Health & Services as Chief Mission Integration Officer. She is the MLC Director of System Integration Initiatives.

William McCready, PhD, has been consulting with the Ministry Leadership Center almost from the beginning to develop measurement and analysis tools, and currently focuses on developing and implementing data-driven evaluation and planning. Bill has held academic posts at the University of Chicago and Northern Illinois University, where he directed the Public Opinion Lab. He is the MLC Senior Fellow for Evaluation & Strategic Planning.

Laurence J. O'Connell, PhD, STD, was formerly president and chief executive officer of the Park Ridge Center for Health, Faith, and Ethics in Chicago, and concurrently served as the chief ethics officer of Advocate Health Care System. Earlier he served as vice president of the Catholic Health Association of the United States and as chairman of the Department of Theological Studies at St. Louis University. Larry has lectured widely, both in the United States and abroad, and has published over a hundred articles, reviews, and books in the fields of theology, bioethics, and health care in several languages. Currently, he is a member of the board of trustees of the Catholic Health Association of the United States. During the Clinton administration, he served at the White House as a member of the President's Health Care Task Force. In 1996, he received the Golden Eurydice Award for "his persistent work in organizing structures of bioethical debate and exceptional contributions to the understanding of sound ethical reasoning," awarded by the Danish Minister of Health at the Danish Parliament (co-recipient Prof. Paul Ricouer). He is the founding MLC Executive Director.

Diarmuid Rooney, MS Psych., MTS, D.Soc.Admin., trained as a clinical psychotherapist in St. Vincent's Hospital, Dublin. He co-founded and directed a community-based counseling and psychotherapy center where his behavioral health work included individual and group therapy, facilitation, and organizational consultancy. Most recently, Diarmuid served as regional director of mission formation for Providence Health & Services in Oregon, where he provided organizational leadership to promote cultural transformation. He is the MLC Director of Integrated Formation Initiatives.

John Shea, STD, was a professor of systematic theology and the director of the Doctor of Ministry Program at the University of St. Mary of the Lake, and a research professor at the Institute of Pastoral Studies at Loyola University of Chicago. He also served as the Advocate Healthcare senior scholar in residence at the Park Ridge Center for Health, Faith, and Ethics and taught at the University of Notre Dame and Boston College. Jack has published over seventy articles and twenty books on contemporary theology and spirituality. He is an internationally recognized lecturer. He is the MLC Director of Program & Processes Development.

Mary Anne Sladich-Lantz, MTS, directs the Providence Leadership Formation program for Providence Health & Services and has served as vice president of mission leadership at St. Patrick Hospital in Missoula, Montana. Mary Anne has a background in psychology and sociology with a master's degree in Theological Studies and Personal Spirituality from the Graduate Theological Union in Berkeley, California. She is the MLC Director for Program Integration Initiatives.

Index